CHILDREN WITH CANCER

CHILDREN WITH CANCER

COMMUNICATION AND EMOTIONS

ANNA M. VAN VELDHUIZEN & BOB F. LAST

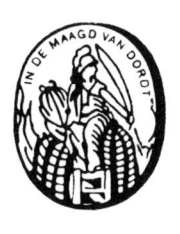

SWETS & ZEITLINGER B.V. AMSTERDAM / LISSE   PUBLISHERS

SWETS & ZEITLINGER INC. ROCKLAND, MA / BERWYN, PA

The study described in this book was funded by a grant from the Dutch Cancer Society and the Foundation for Pediatric Cancer Research.

Library of Congress Cataloging-in-Publication Data

Veldhuizen, Anna M. van 1945-
    Children with cancer : communication and emotions / Anna M. van Veldhuizen, Bob F. Last
    p.   cm.
    Includes bibliographical references.
    Includes index.
    ISBN 9026510381
    1. Tumors in children--Psychological aspects. 2. Tumors in children--Patients--Family relationships. 3. Communication in medicine. 4. Emotions. 5. Adjustment (Psychology) I. Last, Bob F., 1946- . II. Title.
    [DNLM: 1. Communication. 2. Interpersonal Relations. 3. Neoplasms--in infancy & childhood. 4. Neoplasms --psychology.
    QZ 200 V435c]
    RC281.C4V45   1991
    155.9'16--dec20
    DNLM/DLC
    for Library of Congress   90-10213
                                                                                                                                CIP

Cip-gegevens Koninklijke Bibliotheek, Den Haag

Veldhuizen, Anna M. van

Children with cancer : communication and emotions. Anna M. van Veldhuizen & Bob F. Last :[transl. from the Dutch]. - Amsterdam [etc.] : Swets & Zeitlinger. Oorspr. verschenen als proefschrift Universiteit van Amsterdam o.d.t.: Communicatie met het kind met kanker : de wet van de dubbele bescherming. - Amsterdam : Rodopi, 1988. - Met lit. opg.
ISBN 90-265-1038-1
SISO 605.91 UDC 159.9:616-006.6-053.2 NUGI 711
Trefw.: kanker ; kinderen ;psychologie.

Omslagontwerp: Rob Molthof
Druk omslag: Casparie, IJsselstein
Druk: Offsetdrukkerij Kanters B.V., Alblasserdam

© 1991 Swets & Zeitlinger B.V., Amsterdam/Lisse

Alle rechten voorbehouden. Niets uit deze uitgave mag worden verveelvoudigd, opgeslagen in een geautomatiseerd gegevensbestand, of openbaar gemaakt, in enige vorm of op enige wijze, hetzij elektronisch, mechanisch, door fotokopieën, opnamen, of op enige andere manier, zonder voorafgaande schriftelijke toestemming van de uitgever.
Voor zover het maken van kopieën uit deze uitgave is toegestaan op grond van artikel 16B Auteurswet 1912 j° het Besluit van 20 juni 1974 St.b.351, zoals gewijzigd bij het Besluit van 23 augustus 1985, St.b. 471 en artikel 17 Auteurswet 1912, dient men de daarvoor wettelijk verschuldigde vergoedingen te voldoen aan de Stichting Reprorecht (Postbus 882, 1180 AW Amstelveen). Voor het overnemen van gedeelte(n) uit deze uitgave in bloemlezingen, readers en andere compilatiewerken (artikel 16 Auteurswet 1912) dient men zich tot de uitgever te wenden.

All rights reserved. No part of this publication may be reproduced, stored in a retrieval system, or transmitted, in any form or by any means, electronic, mechanical, photocopying, recording, or otherwise, without the prior written permission of the publisher.

ISBN 90 265 1038 1
NUGI 711

Children with Cancer
Anna M. van Veldhuizen and Bob F. Last
© 1991 Amsterdam etc.: SWETS & ZEITLINGER PUBLISHERS

Contents

Introduction	1
1. Childhood cancer: disease, treatment, and prognosis	
1.1. Characteristics of the disease	3
1.2. The incidence of cancer in children	4
1.3. Treatment	4
1.4. Prognosis	8
1.5. Conclusion	11
2. Emotion, stress, and coping	
2.1. The concept of emotion and stress	13
2.2. The situational meaning structure	14
2.3. The concept of coping	18
3. The emotional reactions of the child with cancer and the parents	
3.1. Introduction	25
3.2. The threat to personal concerns	25
3.3. The development of the child's cognitions about emotion	26
3.4. The development of the death concept in children	28
3.5. Awareness of one's own death and fear of death of children with cancer	29
3.6. The situational meaning structure and the emotional reactions of the child	31
3.7. The situational meaning structure and the emotional reactions of the parents	38

4. Communication about the disease
4.1. The concept of communication ... 47
4.2. The function of communication ... 49
4.3. The function of communication about the disease for the child with cancer and the parents ... 54
4.4. Empirical research into the communication processes of children with cancer ... 61
4.5. Empirical research into the relationship between communication about the disease and emotional reactions of children with cancer and their parents ... 63
4.6. Recapitulation ... 67

5. Research design and instruments
5.1. Theoretical framework and the question of the study ... 71
5.2. The research method ... 72
5.3. The instruments ... 76
5.4. The statistical procedures ... 103

6. Test of the hypotheses
6.1. The relationship between the parents' communication style and the child's emotional reactions ... 107
6.2. The relationship between the communication style and the emotional reactions of the parents ... 125

7. Description of the communication process
7.1. Information given by the parents to the child ... 135
7.2. Questions which the child asks the parents about the disease ... 146
7.3. Sources of information, information obstacles, and information needs of the child ... 151
7.4. The parents' attempts at information control ... 160
7.5. Informing the siblings about the disease ... 161
7.6. The parents' information-seeking behavior and their evaluation of information given by the doctor ... 164
7.7. Communication about the emotional experience ... 166
7.8. Communication about the disease in the current stage of the disease ... 173
7.9. The child's knowledge of the disease ... 177

8. Exploration of the intensity of emotional reactions, situational factors and intrapersonal factors
8.1. The intensity of the emotional reactions of the child and the parents ... 181

8.2. The influence of biographical and disease characteristics on the communication style and the emotional
reactions   202
8.3. The child's defensiveness and its relationship with the
emotional reactions of the child and with the
communication style of the parents   221
8.4. The relationship of the communication style with the
coping style and the child-rearing attitudes of
the parents   225

9. Conclusions   231

10. References   241

11. Appendices   253

Introduction

A serious life-threatening disease in a child evokes intense emotions such as fear, grief, despair, and depression. Cancer, cystic fibrosis, muscular dystrophy, severe cardiological and nephrological disorders, and recently also Aids, are diseases which show major differences in the course of the illness and in treatment modalities, but they have one common characteristic: they all threaten the life of the child. Children suffering from such diseases, and their parents too, find themselves in a situation dominated by uncertainty and uncontrollability. In order not to become overpowered by the negative emotions arising from this situation, they have to develop and apply control strategies to reduce uncertainty and uncontrollability. They usually have very few possibilities to change the actual situation and to exercise direct influence on the course of the illness. That is why the child and the parents are forced to appraise the situation in such a way that it will be understandable, acceptable, and endurable for them. Communication about the disease is an important means to reach this goal. The function of communication is the development, maintenance, or alteration of the appraisal which forms the basis of emotions. Communication about the disease also offers the opportunity to express emotions and to find emotional and social support.

In the literature on the emotional consequences of disease and treatment, communication is considered to be an important factor which influences the emotional experience of children and parents. A lesser or greater degree of openness in communication may be practised towards the child with cancer. Open communication about the disease means informing the child about the diagnosis and the prognosis and exchanging information about the emotional experience. Opinions differ on the issue whether open communication has a beneficial influence on emotional experience. On the one hand, there is the opinion that open communication about the disease leaves the child room to express worries and fears, and to seek understanding and support from others. On the other hand, there is the opinion that it is better to protect the child from confrontation with the life-threatening nature of the disease because it would be too much of a burden for a child. Until the beginning of the seventies, childhood cancer almost always had a fatal outcome. Openly informing the child at that time meant the announcement of impending death, an announcement which many understandably recoiled from. With the introduction of more effective treatment methods came the prospect of curing the child with cancer. Since then, openly informing the child about the disease can be combined with giving hope. However, this change in prospect did not generate a routine practice of openly informing the child about the diagnosis and prognosis. The desirability of open communication with the child who has cancer is still under discussion. The few studies conducted on the relation between communication and the emotional experience of child and parents do not provide convincing empirical evidence for either opinion. Moreover, research focuses to a large extent on informing the child. Other aspects of communication such as the verbal and non-verbal exchange of information about the emotional experience and the degree to which the disease is discussed during the rest of the disease period, have hardly ever been studied. The lack of empirical data is probably one of the reasons why a clinical policy in the domain of communication with the child with cancer has not been developed in many hospitals to date. As a result of the absence of a clinical policy, doctors, nurses, and other hospital staff do not follow a common course of behavior in their communication with the child. Another consequence is that sound advice on the best way to communicate with the child can barely be given to the parents, so that they must manage without support in this area.

In this book we report the findings of a study on the communication between parents and their child with cancer. When a child is seriously ill, parents fulfill a key role in the acquisition of information about the disease and in communication about the emotional experience of the disease. Especially young children are highly dependent on their parents for their appraisal of the situation and for emotional support, but older children also rely on their parents if they are stricken with a serious disease. In our study we do not restrict the concept of communication to the information transfer of facts about the disease. The concept also includes the exchange of information on emotions and the degree to which the disease is discussed.

1. Childhood cancer: disease, treatment, and prognosis

1.1. Characteristics of the disease

The group of diseases collectively called cancer is characterized by an uncontrolled and unrestrained proliferation of cells. It may occur as a solid tumor which can spread (metastasize) or as leukemia (cancer of the blood). The different types of cancer are distinguished by the organ and the type of tissue in which the cells are proliferating. Voûte (1985) provides a survey of typical forms of cancer in adults and children. Carcinoma occurs most frequently in adults, starting from the outer tissue layers, the ectoderm. Some types of cancer which primarily develop in adults are: lung carcinoma, stomach carcinoma, mammary carcinoma, bladder carcinoma, and cervical carcinoma. Carcinoma does not often occur in children. Typical malignancies occurring in childhood are sarcoma and blastoma. Sarcoma is a malignant growth of connective tissue. Names of this type of tumor are, for example: osteosarcoma and Ewing's sarcoma (bone tumors), rhabdomyosarcoma (tumor of the muscle tissue), and fibrosarcoma (tumor of connective tissue). A blastoma develops from embryonic tissue, from blastema which is present in each immature organ. Examples of this type of tumor are: nephroblastoma or Wilms' tumor (kidney tumor), hepatoblastoma (liver tumor), medulloblastoma (brain tumor), and neuroblastoma (tumor of the sympathetic nervous system). Besides the previously mentioned malignancies, tumors can also occur in the lymph system, such as Hodgkin's disease and lymphosarcoma. The group of malignant neoplasms in bone marrow and blood, called leukemia, is also a type of cancer. In children, acute lymphocytic leukemia is the most prevalent. If cell proliferation of a tumor or leukemia cannot be stopped, and it displaces healthy tissue and organs and causes loss of function of vital processes, the disease is terminal. Considering current knowledge about the cause of cancer, the following etiological factors play a role: congenital chromosomal defects, ionized radiation, certain chemical substances, and possibly even viruses (Behrendt, 1980; Voûte, 1985; De Waard, 1983). This leads to the paradoxical situation that procedures which must be used to fight cancer – radiation therapy and cytostatics – themselves have carcinogenic properties which could result in the development of a second tumor or leukemia (Behrendt, 1980; Li, 1977; Pinkel, 1980; Voûte, 1985; De Waard, 1983).

1.2. The incidence of cancer in children

Cancer is a relatively rare disease in children. Because there is no complete registration yet of malignant disorders in children in the Netherlands, incidence rates must still be based on estimates. It is estimated that, in the Netherlands, the incidence of childhood cancer is 1 per 10,000 children a year between the ages of 0 and 17. This means 400 new cases per year (Voûte, 1985). Registration of children with leukemia does exist on a nationwide level in the Netherlands. Research by Van Steensel-Moll (1983) shows that an annual average of 108 children in the Netherlands between the ages of 0 and 15 are diagnosed as having leukemia. For the age group 0 to 18, it is estimated that leukemia constitutes 30–35% of the malignancies in childhood (Sjamsoedin-Visser & Van Leeuwen, 1983). Leukemia occurs somewhat more often among boys than among girls. Van Steensel-Moll (1983) found a sex ratio of 1:2. Other types of cancer are also encountered more often among boys than among girls (Koocher, 1981). Furthermore, the different types of cancer are not distributed equally among the different age groups. Leukemia usually develops in children between the third and fifth year (Van Steensel-Moll, 1983). Blastomas, such as neuroblastoma and Wilms' tumor, also usually appear in younger children, while sarcomas such as osteosarcoma, Ewing's sarcoma, and rhabdomyosarcoma are more prevalent among older children and adolescents (Voûte, 1985).

1.3. Treatment

The same treatment modalities are applied in the therapy of childhood cancer as in the therapy of cancer in adults, i.e. surgery, radiotherapy, and chemotherapy. Usually different treatment modalities are combined. Chemotherapeutic agents consist of many kinds of cytostatics (cell-growth inhibitors and cell-killing agents). Cytostatics are usually administered in different combinations. In the Netherlands, just like in the rest of Europe and the United States, most children with cancer are treated in specialized centers. The Netherlands has four Children's Oncology Centers, one of which is located in the Emma Kinder Ziekenhuis in Amsterdam. The tentative diagnosis is usually made elsewhere and sometimes treatment is initiated there before the child is referred to a Children's Oncology Center for further diagnostic examination and treatment. In the Children's Oncology Center in Amsterdam in the period 1975 till 1985, an average of 97 children (from 0–18 years) were admitted annually for (further) diagnostic examination and treatment. More than three-quarters of the children (77%) had a tumor and almost one-quarter (23%) had leukemia (based on data from the registration of the Children's Tumor Workgroup Amsterdam).

The precise nature and duration of the treatment are dependent on the type of cancer, its location, the degree of growth and spread of the tumor, and other prognostic factors. Whether treatment is entirely or mainly given in hospital, or whether it can be outpatient treatment also depends on treatment intensity and the occurrence of complications. On the basis of clinical research, treatment schedules are changed and adjusted regularly. In the Children's Oncology Center in Amsterdam, as in most other centers, children with acute lymphocytic leukemia are treated in three stages. Induction therapy is followed by a prophylactic therapy of the central nervous system (CNS-prophylaxis) and a maintenance therapy for an extended period of time. The induction therapy takes place in hospital or is given as day care treatment. It generally lasts 6 to 10 weeks. Several types of cytostatics are administered, including high doses of methotrexate. CNS-prophylaxis is necessary to prevent spread of leukemic cells to the meninges. In the recent past, CNS-prophylaxis consisted of cranial radiotherapy, but since 1984 this form of treatment has been replaced in the Netherlands by high doses of methotrexate and prolonged administering of intrathecal cytostatics to avoid the harmful effects of radiotherapy on the child's neuropsychological functioning (Lansky et al., 1984; Last et al., 1982a; Meadows et al., 1981; Moss et al., 1981). It has been proven that the same treatment results can be achieved by this more intensive general treatment (Behrendt, 1984). Nowadays cranial radiotherapy is only given in cases of CNS relapse or high risk of CNS relapse. The maintenance therapy usually lasts one and a half to two years. In this stage of treatment, the child has to take cytostatics orally everyday, and has to visit the clinic frequently for physical examination and blood tests. Cytotstatics are also administered there intravenously to some of the patients. Moreover, the child gets bone marrow aspirations and lumbar punctures every three months to evaluate whether there is continuous remission (absence of disease symptoms) or relapse (recurrence of disease symptoms). The treatment programs for other forms of leukemia are generally shorter, but more intensive. The chemotherapeutic treatment is sometimes followed by allogeneic or autologous bone marrow transplantation. Autologous bone marrow transplantations are performed in the Children's Oncology Center in Amsterdam.

As in the treatment of leukemia, new developments in the treatment of tumors in children can sometimes prevent serious side effects and mutilations resulting from the treatment (Voûte, 1985). The treatment of osteosarcoma, usually located in the leg, is an example of this. Besides intensive chemotherapy, it is almost always necessary to amputate the child's limb. Due to the availability of new cytostatics and combination chemotherapy, it is now possible in some cases to reduce the tumor to such an extent that local resection can be carried out and thus the limb can be saved. In general, treatment of tumors consists of removal of the tumor, if possible. Initial surgery (biopsy or removal of the tumor) is sometimes performed in the hospital to which the child was initially referred. If the tumor was not removed completely, then the child can again undergo surgery in the Children's Oncology Center. Cytostatic therapy is usually included in the treatment, and sometimes radiotherapy is applied to the tumor area and/or the areas where metastases have occurred. Metastases in the lungs are preferably removed surgically, because radiotherapy can result in severe loss of pulmonary functioning.

The mode and duration of treatment depend on the type of tumor, the stage of the disease (e.g. determined by the size of the tumor and/or the degree of metastasizing), and the effectiveness of the previous treatment. Some examples of treatment schedules used in the Children's Oncology Center in Amsterdam are shown in Table 1.1.

If, after initial cytostatic treatment and/or surgery and/or radiotherapy, treatment continues on an outpatient basis, the number of hospitalizations and days in hospital can be kept at a minimum for the child. The frequency of administering cytostatic drugs to the child varies from 1 x per 14 days to 1 x per 6 weeks. During the administration of cytostatics in hospital (possibly in combination with administering during visits to the clinic), the child stays in hospital each time for a few days (2-10). The total number of hospitalizations, per child, can therefore amount to a few dozen and the total number of days in hospital to well over a hundred. In case of

Table 1.1
Treatment schedules for various types of tumors

Type of tumor	Nature of the treatment				Duration of treatment in months
	Chemotherapy		Radiotherapy	Surgery	
	Hospitali-zation	Out-patient			
Hodgkin's disease:					
stage I and II		x			6
stage III and IV	x	x			6
Medulloblastoma	x		x	x	4
Osteosarcoma	x			x	3-5
Ewing's sarcoma	x	x	(x)	(x)	12
Wilms' tumor:					
stage I and II	x	x		x	12
stage III and IV	x	x	x	x	12
Rhabdomyosarcoma	x	x	(x)	(x)	6-18
Lymphosarcoma	x	x		(x)	6-18

x = type of treatment used for the majority of patients
(x) = type of treatment which varies greatly for different patients

severe complications, the child will usually have to be admitted to the hospital as well. For both leukemia and tumors, the treatment is intensified if there is a relapse or recurrence, or if the treatment has insufficient effect. An intensified treatment is started again if a relapse or recurrence occurs after treatment has been terminated.

Due to the many and sometimes severe side effects of cytostatics, and due to the mutilating operations which are sometimes necessary, cancer treatment is labelled 'aggressive'. The severity of the side effects of surgery is determined by the loss of functioning of the organ removed (eye, kidney, arm, or leg) and by the possible damage to other tissues or organs which may have occurred during surgery. The side effects of cytostatics and radiotherapy can reinforce one another if both therapies are used together (Jaffe et al., 1981).

Cytostatics have a number of general and a number of specific toxic side effects (Behrendt, 1984; Boogaerts & Dekker, 1983; Sjamsoedin-Visser & Van Leeuwen, 1983; Voûte, 1985). The most prevalent temporary side effects are bone marrow aplasia, nausea, vomiting, loss of appetite, infection of mucous membrane, alopecia, skin irritations, and sensory and motor disorders. Permanent effects which could arise as side effects of cytostatics are kidney and liver damage, damage to the heart muscle, neurological damage, loss of hearing, loss of pulmonary function, and, in some cases, infertility and a second malignancy (Dobkin & Morrow, 1985). The temporary bone marrow aplasia (arrest or highly restrained growth of healthy blood cells) which occurs when high doses of cytostatics are administered, results in the danger of life-threatening infections or haemorrhages. Infection is still the most common cause of death during remission-induction therapy (Boogaerts & Dekker, 1983). During the occurrence of a bone marrow aplasia, it is necessary to nurse the child in an isolation ward to decrease the risk of infection. A diminished immunity against infections remains during the entire period of cytostatic therapy and even a few months after termination of treatment. Because children have often developed insufficient immunity against viruses, there is great danger that a life-threatening infection from certain viruses such as chicken pox can occur (Sjamsoedin-Visser & Van Leeuwen, 1983).

Temporary side effects of cranial radiotherapy are alopecia, fatigue, nausea, and vomiting (Behrendt, 1980). For children, radiotherapy on bones (face, spinal column, limbs) can result in permanently reduced growth which causes deformities (Jaffe et al., 1981; Voûte, 1985). Cranial radiotherapy given to children with leukemia can result in a slow decline of growth rate (Sjamsoedin-Visser & Van Leeuwen, 1983). For children with a brain tumor, cranial radiotherapy can be partially responsible for the cessation of the production of growth hormones and/or other hypophyseal hormones (Voûte, 1985). Neuropsychological changes as a result of cranial radiotherapy such as declines in intelligence, and concentration and learning disabilities, have been observed in children with leukemia (Eiser & Lansdown, 1977; Lansky et al., 1984; Last et al., 1982a; Meadows et al., 1981; Moss et al., 1981; Rowland et al., 1984). Besides permanent organ damage and loss of functions, radiotherapy increases the chance of development of a second tumor or leukemia (Dobkin & Morrow, 1985; Li, 1977).

1.4. Prognosis

In (pediatric) oncology it is not possible to establish with any certainty whether a patient is cured. Clinical methods are lacking for determining whether all cancer cells have been destroyed, after termination of therapy. The risk of relapse or recurrence can therefore never be ruled out (Behrendt, 1984; Pinkel, 1980). Thus treatment results are usually expressed in terms of survival rates or disease-free survival rates. At the end of the '60's and the beginning of the '70's, treatment results for children with cancer have become considerably more favorable. Before that time, leukemia in children almost always followed a fatal course. The average survival duration was usually only a few months (Behrendt, 1984; Romsdahl, 1980). The treatment results of children with tumors were somewhat more promising at that time. For all children with cancer in the United States, the five-year survival at the end of the '50's and the beginning of the '60's was 30% (Romsdahl, 1980). These results are probably close to the treatment results which were achieved in the Netherlands. However, precise data on this are lacking. Even now, national data on treatment results of children with cancer are still not available in the Netherlands. Although survival rates vary according to diagnosis, in recent American literature a five-year survival of about 50% is reported for both the total group of children with cancer and for children with acute lymphocytic leukemia (Van

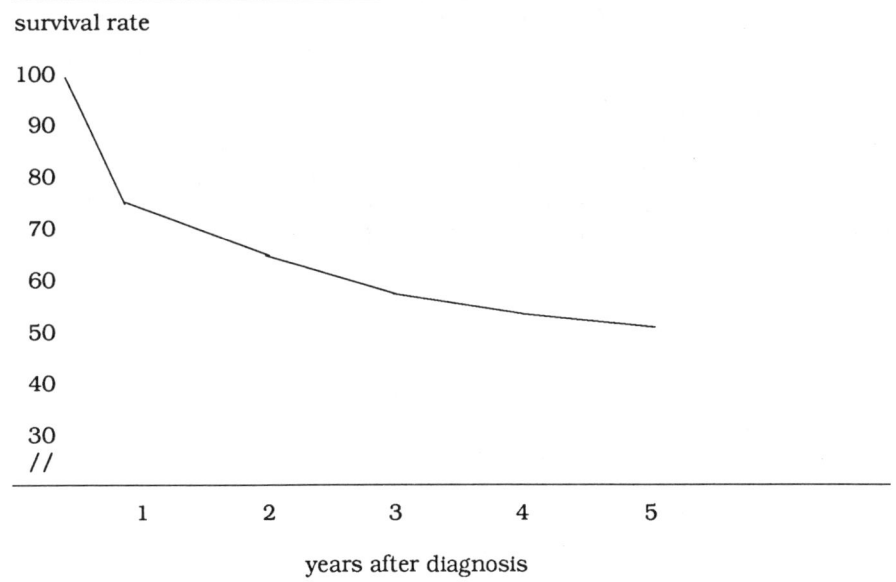

Figure 1.1
Five-year survival curve of the total group of children with cancer (0-18 years) in the period 1974 to 1982, admitted for initial therapy to the Children's Oncology Center in Amsterdam, n = 745. (based on data from the registration of the Children's Tumor Workgroup Amsterdam).

Eys & Sullivan, 1980; George, 1980). Treatment results achieved at the Children's Oncology Center in Amsterdam correspond with this. In Figure 1.1 it appears that mortality is highest in the first and second year after diagnosis. In the following years, the mortality rate decreases greatly. Five years after diagnosis, 52% of the children are still alive. The five-year survival is almost equivalent for children with tumors and for children with leukemia. After five years, 53% of the children with a tumor and 52% of the children with leukemia are still alive. If we make a distinction for leukemia between acute lymphocytic leukemia and other types of leukemia, then the five-year survival is 64% for children with acute lymphocytic leukemia and 13% for children with other types of leukemia.

Not only in the case of leukemia does the prognosis strongly correspond with the type of leukemia, but also in the case of tumors there are large differences in prognosis, depending on the type of tumor. Children with a Wilms' tumor and Hodgkin's disease generally have a better prognosis than children with neuroblastoma or a brain tumor (Siegel, 1980; Voûte et al., 1980). The prognosis is further determined by the stage of the disease or the degree of spread at the time of diagnosis, by specific diagnostic characteristics of the disease, and sometimes also by the child's age (Behrendt, 1984; George, 1980; Pinkel, 1980). A relapse or recurrence nearly always means a considerable deterioration of the survival chances.

Progress in treatment results makes it possible to study the survival duration of children with cancer over a longer period of time. Regarding the total group of children with cancer, Li et al. (1978) proved that five years after diagnosis one still cannot say with certainty that a cure has been effected. Of the children in the group they studied, who were still alive five years after diagnosis, 8% died of a relapse or recurrence in the following years and 1% of the children died of a second primary tumor. The long-term prognosis turned out to be much better if no relapse or recurrence had occurred in the first five years after diagnosis. The mortality rate as a result of relapse or recurrence was highest 5 to 10 years after diagnosis, while the mortality rate as a result of a second primary tumor was highest 10 to 15 years after diagnosis. The group studied by Li et al. consisted of children treated between 1947 and 1969. Methods of treatment have changed since then. However, for the group of children with cancer who were admitted for initial therapy to the Children's Oncology Center in Amsterdam between 1974 to 1977 and who were treated according to new treatment protocols, it could also be established that between the fifth and tenth year after diagnosis, an average of 1% of the children with a tumor and

3% of the children with acute lymphocytic leukemia died of a relapse or recurrence each year.

1.5. Conclusion

The advances of medical treatment for cancer in children make this disease more difficult to define and classify. The disease used to be categorized under acute diseases. It had a predictable and quickly fatal course: remission, relapse or recurrence, death. The prolonged survival now attained by many children is the reason for presently classifying cancer in children as a chronic illness. Comaroff and Maguire (1981) correctly point out that this division is problematic. The most salient characteristic of the disease now is the unpredictability of its course and final outcome. More knowledge of prognostic factors provides statistical knowledge, but this does not have very much bearing on individual cases. After a favorable course of treatment, at each check-up, the doctor can only say that everything is going well for the moment. Like every acute illness, cancer is still acutely life-threatening and for a number of children the disease still follows an acute course. The mortality rate is highest in the first year after diagnosis (see Figure 1.1). For a relatively large number of children it now applies that new treatment methods do slow down a fatal course, but they do not prevent it. Moreover, there is no clearly definable stage in which it can be said that the disease is being controlled or that the crisis has been overcome. The term remission is ambiguous, both in a clinical sense and in the experience of those involved. It can mean both the absence or the latent presence of disease symptoms. Positive certainty about a cure cannot be given. The longer a child remains in remission the better the child's chances are, but a relapse or recurrence can still occur at any time. The fact that the presence of latent cancer cells cannot be ruled out makes cancer a chronic illness. But the question remains how realistic it is to label a child, who has not exhibited any physical complaints or disease symptoms for many years, as a chronically ill child. Permanent damage as a result of the disease or treatment which hinders normal functioning would sooner lead to the child being labelled as handicapped than as chronically ill. What can be called chronic is the permanent threat and the long-term period of uncertainty.

2. Emotion, stress and coping

2.1. The concept of emotion and stress

Emotions are often indicated as a state of a person. However, emotions are not static but are events which continually change over time. Frijda (1986) defines emotions as changes in action readiness leading to an emotional response that consists of a physiological reaction, an experiential reaction, and behavior. We use Frijda's emotion theory as the starting point for a description of the situation and of the emotional reactions which this situation arouses in the child with cancer and in the parents. His theory is a specification and an integration of cognitive theories on stress and emotion (Arnold, 1960; Lazarus, 1966; Mandler, 1975). In these theories, stress is interpreted as a cognitive psychological construct, in contradistinction to the first researchers of human and animal stress.

Stress was initially described as a physiological concept. Selye (1956), the most important proponent of this approach, defined stress as 'the condition which manifests itself as a specific reaction pattern and consists of all changes created within a biological system by non-specific factors'. Selye uses the concept of stress as the indicator of a response pattern. The specific responses are aroused by stimuli which are called stressors. Research into stress symptoms as a response refers to physiological reaction patterns. An example of this is the study on the enhanced secretion of a stress-related hormone in parents of children with leukemia (Hofer et al., 1972; Wolff et al., 1964).

In the traditional stimulus-response approach to stress, emphasis is placed on the influence of prominent events in someone's personal life (serious life events), on the ability to adapt, and on the individual's state of health (Holmes & Rahe, 1967; Rahe, 1974). It is characteristic of the later 'serious life events' research that the models become more complex and the role of informational and cognitive processes have been included in the models (Horowitz, 1979). In recent approaches stress is conceptualized as the result of an interaction between the individual and the environment. Nothing is stressful unless the individual interprets it as such. In this view, stress is defined as a relationship between the individual and the environment, where the environment is evaluated by the individual as threatening to his or her well-being, and in which the environmental demands tax or exceed the resources of the person (Lazarus & Folkman, 1984). Thus perception and evaluation of a situation take a central position in this approach. As an indicator of this perceptual and evaluational process, Lazarus (1966) uses the term 'appraisal'. Every person evaluates each stimulus. A situation can be interpreted as irrelevant, good, or harmful. The cognitive process of interpretation precedes the emotion. Three appraisal processes are distinguished here. Primary appraisal is the evaluation of the importance of the situation for personal well-being. Secondary appraisal refers to whether the individual can do something about the situation. And finally, reappraisal concerns the changes in evaluation as a result of changes in the situation, which could partly be the result of the person's own actions. This last aspect of the appraisal process indicates the continuous interaction between the individual and the environment, in which the result of one's own coping efforts to influence the situation is involved in the evaluation (Folkman et al., 1979; Lazarus & Folkman, 1984; Lazarus & Launier, 1978). Lazarus and Folkman (1984) use a transactional model to define stress in order to accentuate, among other things, the dynamic reciprocal relationship between the individual and the environment. In his emotion theory, Frijda (1986) provides a detailed analysis of the cognitive processes which are involved in emotions. He uses the concept of situational meaning structure to indicate these cognitive processes.

2.2. The situational meaning structure

Emotions can be considered as psychological reactions to events which are relevant for the concerns of a person (Frijda, 1986). The term concern here indicates the dispositions which motivate a person to avoid, seek, or further certain events. Events which correspond to what the individual desires (safety, absence of pain, self-esteem, being liked) evoke positive emotions. Events which do not correspond to the needs or desires of the individual (pain, rejection, loss of a loved one) evoke negative emotions. A person's concerns can be characterized as dispositions which are latently present and only become manifest if events take place which damage or threaten to damage a desire, or which satisfy or promise to satisfy a desire. Health is important for a person who becomes ill. It is only then that health get its full share of attention. The child's concern for the mother's presence becomes noticeable when she leaves. The young child attempts to follow her, expresses the desire for her to remain, and gets upset if this wish is not fulfilled. Therefore events must be relevant to the individual's concerns before they cause an emotional reaction. To which emotion these events lead is determined by the situational meaning structure. Frijda distinguishes three elements in the situational meaning structure:

> Cognitions of what the situation does or offers to the subject or withholds from him, or might do or offer or withhold.
> Cognitions of what the situation allows him to do, prevents him from doing, or invites him to do.
> Cognitions of whether the various outcomes are desirable or not.

In his theory, Frijda provides an analysis of the components of the situational meaning structure. Various components explain why and when a certain emotion will arise, why there are transitions between emotions over time, and why there are similarities between emotions. Each emotion consists of a pattern of components. Similarities between emotions arise in part from common components, and transitions between emotions occur when the person's attention is directed towards other components of the situation. In the following sections we will describe those components which probably play an important role in the appraisal of the situation by the child who has cancer, and the parents.

Responsibility for the situation

For emotions such as anger, guilt, and pride to arise, it is necessary to hold someone responsible for the situation in which one finds oneself. Although nothing or no one can be held responsible for the onset of cancer in the child, there is still the need to put the blame on someone or something. This enables anger to be directed somewhere and, at the least, can serve as a temporary attribution of guilt. Thus the doctor can become the object of anger as the bearer of the bad news. Together with the nursing staff, the doctor can also be considered as one who inflicts pain and who is the instigator of a treatment which makes the child feel very ill. The family doctor can be held responsible for not recognizing the usually vague symptoms of the disease on time, since early diagnosis and treatment are so important for the survival chances of the child. The pediatrician can become the object of anger if it finally becomes apparent that, in spite of his or her expertise, he or she fails to cure the child. Besides the doctor, a higher power such as God or Fate can also be blamed for causing this situation. The young child can direct his or her anger at the parents if the child holds the parents responsible for leaving him or her behind in the hospital and for not offering protection against pain and grief (Bowlby, 1973). If a person does not see something or someone else but him or herself as the cause of the situation, then feelings of guilt can arise, or pride as a positive variant. Thus parents can blame themselves for having waited too long before bringing the child to the family doctor or for not having insisted on referral to a pediatrician. The child can consider the disease and the stay in hospital as punishment for norm-violating behavior. On the other hand, both the child and the parents can experience feelings of pride if they partly attribute the success of the treatment to their own efforts and endurance, in spite of all the difficulties.

Controllability and uncontrollability of the situation

When a situation is considered to be controllable, this constitutes an important component for a person's feelings of security, confidence, competence, and power. However, when a situation is seen as uncontrollable, this creates a condition for anxiety and fear (Averill, 1973; Lazarus et al., 1980) and for helplessness and depression (Seligman, 1975). A disease such as cancer creates a situation which is dominated by uncontrollability. Technical progress attained in medical science in the past decades makes the limited knowledge of the etiology and the relatively limited possibilities for controlling this disease glaringly obvious. The disease process does not have clearly defined stages in which a complete control or cure of the disease can be guaranteed. Furthermore, the potential control of the disease process is mainly in the hands of the doctor. Children and parents cannot influence the disease process very much. Moreover, parents must entrust most of the care of their child to others in the hospital. They must also witness how their child is exposed to 'pathogenic' treatment and painful procedures. The child too has very little influence on the events which emanate from the disease and the treatment. But the absence of actual control of the situation does not mean that child and parents are unable to reduce their feelings of anxiety and helplessness. The idea and the feeling of being able to exercise some control of the situation and not only being an unwilling victim, can be sufficient to reduce negative emotions (Averill, 1973; Rothbaum et al., 1982).

Certainty and uncertainty about the situation

The consequences of an event which has not yet occurred, or not entirely, are uncertain. They do not have to take place; they could still be averted. Anticipation of the consequences of a future event is an important component in eliciting emotions such as fear and hope. Fear and hope imply uncertain outcomes. There is doubt about the future. With increasing certainty of a negative outcome, fear is transformed into despair. With increasing certainty of a favorable outcome, hope is transformed into confidence. Due to the unpredictability of the course of the illness and the long-term uncertainty about the final outcome, the child and parents find themselves in a situation between hope and fear. The anticipated threat of a fatal outcome hangs above their head like a 'sword of Damocles' (Koocher & O'Malley, 1981). From the moment that the first symptoms of a serious illness manifest themselves in the child, numerous uncertainties arise. Prior to the diagnosis, there is the uncertainty whether the terrible suspicion will be confirmed. After the diagnosis there is uncertainty about the prognosis, the length and severity of the treatment, the length and number of hospital admissions, the side effects of therapy on the well-being and development of the child, the complications which could arise, and the test results which could indicate a remission or, on the contrary, a relapse or recurrence of the disease. The degree to which these events are anticipated and become conditions for fear or hope depends, on the one hand, on the information and/or the knowledge, based on experience, which one has of the probability of these events, and depends, on the other hand, on the subjective meaning which is attributed to objective (statistical) probabilities. De Swaan (1982) summarizes this process for adult cancer patients as follows:

> "The precise data which are available on the disease are of secondary importance. Even if the patient knows that nine out of ten persons die of this particular disease, why should he or she not be the tenth? And: Even if only one of the ten persons dies of this disease, who can guarantee that he or she will not be that one?" (pp. 193-194).

Fluctuations between emotions of hope and fear can be the result of a confrontation with a succession of alternating hopeful and fear-inducing events, or of attention shifts between positive and negative aspects of an event.

Restriction of freedom of action

Restriction of freedom of action is dominant in situations which lead to anger, frustration, disappointment, and loneliness. Physical limitations as a result of the disease are present for the child in many situations, and thus also for the parents who are entrusted with the child's care. Hospital admission, confinement to bed, being nursed on an isolation ward, clinic visits, inability to participate in certain sports (e.g. after an amputation), having to remain at home, and being unable to attend school, are examples of situations in which freedom of actions are considerably restricted. Physical restrictions result, directly or indirectly, in social isolation and thus constitute an important component in the development of feelings of loneliness. For both the child and the parents, there are fewer opportunities for taking part in activities, independently or together. There are also fewer opportunities to socialize with others outside the family. Other persons are seen, to a greater or lesser extent, as physically and psychologically unattainable. The result can be that they are blamed for not understanding the situation. On the other hand, people could start avoiding the family. The child's illness can lead to stigmatizing the family (Goffman, 1963).

The long duration of the situation

Feelings of depression especially arise in situations where persons feel they have little control over the outcomes of their actions and also do not expect that this will be the case in future (Seligman, 1975). Besides this expectation, previous experience with long-term negative stimulus conditions over which no control is felt to be had can also cause feelings of gloom. The treatment schedules for children with cancer cover a period of 4 months to 2 years (see section 1.3). If there is a recurrence or relapse, the length of treatment is considerably extended. This means that the child and the parents must undergo the restrictions and discomforts of the severe treatments for a long period. Besides the length of treatment, the length of time elapsed since diagnosis is also important. We have already said that even a period of many years of disease-free survival still does not mean the absolute certainty of being cured. The long duration of the stressful situation can create a condition of exhaustion and gloom for child and parents because, as stated, they can exert little or no influence here. On the other hand, the experience of a long period of absence of disease symptoms can increase confidence in a positive outcome and reinforce feelings of hope.

2.3. The concept of coping

How a person deals with stressful situations is called coping. Coping is related to psychological concepts such as adaptation, mastery, and defense mechanisms (White, 1974). In recent approaches to stress, coping is becoming increasingly important. The degree to which someone is successful in mastering a difficult situation determines the degree to which the situation is evaluated and experienced as stressful. In studies on the development and use of coping strategies, several different strategies can be distinguished. Some researchers consider coping to be a personality trait. Coping behavior is considered here to be a stable trait of a person which has developed on the basis of previous learning experiences associated with existing dispositions. This approach results in a distinction between types of behavior which differentiate individuals, for example, as repressors or sensitizers (Byrne, 1964), as monitors or blunters (Miller, 1980), or as persons using approach behavior or avoidance behavior, which is how Lowenberg (1970) differentiates parents of fatally ill children. Coping behavior related to heart diseases is described as type A behavior (Glass, 1977a, 1977b). Type A persons are characterized, as having a strong commitment to control situations. When control is threatened or frustrated, they become highly emotional, strive excessively to strengthen control, and feel desperate if they do not succeed. Individuals with this personality trait are vulnerable and experience extreme stress reactions under conditions which allow few opportunities for control. The disadvantage of defining coping behavior as a personality trait is that it implies a stable reaction pattern which cannot easily be adjusted if this is required by the situation (Singer, 1984). Thus other researchers prefer to describe coping behavior as a style. A coping style indicates a relatively stable reaction pattern for persons in difficult situations but, depending on the specific situation, it also implies a certain flexibility (Schreurs et al., 1986a). According to these researchers, it is possible to modify coping behavior. In a study of surgical patients, it was proven that altering coping behavior can be achieved by short-term counselling (Janis, 1985). Lazarus and Folkman (1984) go further and consider coping to be a transactional process between the person and the environment. They define coping as 'constantly changing cognitive and behavioral efforts to manage specific external and/or internal demands that are appraised as taxing or exceeding the resources of the person'. Although in the view of coping as a process a certain consistency in the individual's reaction pattern is not ruled out, the emphasis lies on the ongoing interaction between the person and the environment. On the basis of the individual's reaction to the situation, new evaluations (reappraisals) are made which lead to new reactions.

The function of coping

In dealing with stressful situations, two forms of coping can be distinguished. First, reactions aimed at controlling the difficult situation, locating the causes of the difficult situation, and changing these or removing them. These strategies are called problem-focused methods of coping (Lazarus & Folkman, 1984). Second, reactions aimed at regulating the emotions which arise because of the difficult situation. These reactions are not intended to alter the objective situation, but serve to reduce the increased arousal level caused by the stressful circumstances. These strategies are called emotion-focused methods of coping.

Problem-focused coping. Problem-focused coping is related to defining the problem, generating alternative solutions, weighing alternatives in terms of their costs and benefits, choosing among them, and acting. All these actions can be seen as attempts at primary control of the situation, namely adjusting the situation to suit one's wishes (Rothbaum et al., 1982). For cancer patients these attempts at primary control of the situation, or rather controlling the course of the illness, are often very extreme. They consist of (persisting in) seeking medical help, undergoing and accepting the strongly aversive consequences of therapy, and persistence in attempting to change the situation, even if the efforts seem useless and cannot halt the disease process. The persistence for primary control of the situation originates from one overpowering desire: the desire to live. Giving up or abandoning attempts to control the disease means death. If such a fate can be accepted at all, it can only be accepted by the patient, family, and the doctors after a long, exhausting struggle.

Rothbaum et al. (1982) distinguish various types of primary control: predictive, illusory, vicarious, and interpretative control. These types of problem-focused coping can be used by the child with cancer and the parents. They can seek information about the disease, the treatment programs, and about conventional and unorthodox forms of therapy in an attempt to understand their situation and to promote possible solutions (interpretative control). With knowledge of the expected course of the illness, the treatment schedule, and the side effects of therapy, they can predict events and enhance control (predictive control). Attempts to influence the chance-determined outcome of the illness can be sought for in changes in lifestyle and eating habits (illusory control). The solution to the problem, i.e. control of the disease process, cannot be realized by the child or the parents themselves but must be entrusted to the doctor. But they can attempt to influence the doctor's choices when establishing, continuing, altering, or terminating therapy (vicarious control). These attempts are usually not made often during the initial stage of the disease because patient and parents realize their dependence on the experience and expertise of the doctor, but these attempts increase if it becomes apparent that the doctor's expertise to control the disease is insufficient. The child and more often the parents attempt to convince the doctor in this stage to continue treatment, to even consider the use of experimental drugs and therapies. For that matter, usually not much persuasion is necessary to motivate the doctor to continue, because it's also difficult for the doctor to accept that his or her attempts have failed and the child will die. It has already been stated that the possibilities for controlling a disease such as cancer are limited and the outcome is uncertain. Due to this, the child and the parents have to rely heavily on secondary control strategies.

Emotion-focused coping. All actions which serve to diminish negative emotions are categorized as emotion-focused coping (Lazarus & Folkman, 1984). These actions mainly consist of cognitive processes. Emotion-focused coping is related to Rothbaum's et al. (1982) concept of secondary control. If primary control fails or is impossible and the situation cannot be changed, individuals adjust themselves to the situation. The aforementioned types of control (predictive, illusory, vicarious, and interpretative) are also applied in secondary control. By taking the expected negative effects of the treatment into account, and by accepting the worst - a fatal outcome of the disease - child and parents can protect themselves against disappointments (predictive control). They can search for the meaning of the occurrence of the disease: why this has happened to them, and thus attempt to accept their situation (interpretative control). They can take the side of fate, admit that fate is more powerful, but assume that fate will be kind to them (illusory control). This type of control is manifest in parents who ascribe specific traits to their child, such as courage and bravery, so that they differentiate their child as one of the lucky ones who will survive. The child too can count itself as a survivor by demonstrating courage and bravery. Furthermore, child and parents can attribute special power to the doctor, on whom all hope is focused, so that, through the doctor, they can gain control of the situation (vicarious control).

Rothbaum et al. point out that searching for the meaning of events is especially intense under conditions in which minimal opportunities exist for primary control. A considerable amount of energy is invested in interpreting aversive situations because absolute lack of control is highly threatening, and a feeling of control is associated with understanding events and accepting them. In the authors' opinion, interpretative control is intrinsically rewarding and not only a means to achieve positive thoughts and a cheerful mood, although this often results from having found an explanation of the situation. From observations of parents of children with leukemia, Comaroff and Maguire (1981) infer that 'the search for meaning' is most characteristic of the way in which parents cope with the situation. In their search for an explanation of their child's disease, many parents blamed themselves. Feelings of guilt are often observed in victims of disasters, torture, sexual abuse, or child abuse. These feelings of guilt are paradoxical because these victims are in no way responsible for the traumatic events which they were exposed to. Frijda (1987) explains such phenomena by applying the law of minimal loss and maximum gain: when a situation can be viewed in different ways, there is an inclination to look at it in such a way that the emotional burden is minimal and the benefit is greatest. According to Frijda, feelings of guilt are preferable to the greater distress of feeling helpless, and having to accept complete arbitrariness and meaninglessness. It is better to regard oneself as guilty, so that the distress can at least be understood and the illusion of a just world can be maintained. Feelings of guilt give meaning to meaninglessness. This maintains the illusion that the situation can be changed as well as the illusion that one has power over fate. The law of minimal loss and maximum gain applies to all emotions. Like feelings of guilt, anger maintains the illusion that the situation can be changed and undone by those who have caused it; but anger also prevents one from having to resign oneself to an inevitable fate.

The classical defense mechanisms which also belong to emotion-focused forms of coping such as denial, repression, intellectualization, and reaction formation, are especially used by persons exposed to traumatic events. Denial as an initial reaction to learning the diagnosis is often described in parents of children with cancer (Kaplan, 1977; Lowenberg, 1970; Natterson & Knudson, 1960). Denial is considered to be a protective mechanism by which a person gains time to slowly assimilate the facts so as not to become overwhelmed by them. Not only can the threatening information be denied, but also the personal relevance or urgency of the threat, the emotion itself, or the relationship between the emotion and the threat (Breznitz, 1983). Because of the many types of denial and related reactions such as avoidance, Lazarus (1981, 1983) talks about a 'family of denial'. The distinction between denial and avoidance is often difficult to establish. A terminally ill child and the parents can both know that death is closing in, but may prefer not to think about this or discuss it. This is an example of avoidance and not of denial, but for the outsider this remains unclear. There is another ambiguity which especially plays an important role for children with cancer: the child cannot deny what it does not know. If the doctor or the parents have not informed the child of the diagnosis and the prognosis or have done this in a vague manner, then there is no way to determine whether the child does not know it or is denying it. Denial is assumed to be a coping strategy for children with cancer where research results indicate a low degree of anxiety, hope for the future, and concrete future plans (Kellerman et al., 1980; Mulhern et al., 1981; Nannis et al., 1982; Zeltzer et al., 1980).

Hope is an important prerequisite for the motivation to act as well as for the final actions themselves (Stotland, 1969). Hope and optimism concerning the outcome of the disease process are essential for being able to cope with the aversive treatment and promote an adequate adjustment to the disease (Kaplan, 1977; Koocher & O'Malley, 1981; Lowenberg, 1970). Denying the facts can be detrimental in situations requiring direct action (reacting to disease symptoms), but denying the implications of facts (possible or certain fatal outcome) can be beneficial and further optimism (Lazarus, 1981). However, parents who deny the implications for a longer period may have to pay a price. Parents who deny the threatened loss of their child experience a greater shock when the child actually dies and have a more problematic mourning process than parents who have taken the loss of their child into account and show anticipatory grief (Hofer et al., 1972; Townes et al., 1974). Denial and predictive control are each other's opposites. In both cases one wants to be on the safe side. It may not be certain whether the parents will lose the child, but by opting for denial they cling to the notion that the child will surely survive, and by opting for predictive control they prepare themselves for, in their view, the certain death of the child.

3. The emotional reactions of the child with cancer and the parents

3.1. Introduction

In the literature, descriptions of the emotional reactions of children with cancer and their parents are seldom put into a conceptual framework. An exception to this is an article by Van Dongen-Melman et al. (1986) in which the psychosocial functioning of children with cancer and their parents is described employing social-psychological theories (attribution theory and social comparison theory). Much of the literature is based on clinical impressions and insufficiently controlled studies of children and parents. However, objective empirical research has increased in the past few years. In this chapter, we present a review of descriptive studies and empirical research on the emotional reactions of children with cancer and their parents. Literature on other (serious) diseases in children is included here. For the description of the emotional reactions, we will use Frijda's (1986) emotion theory as a starting point. Within this theoretical framework we assume the emotional reactions to be the result of information processing and the outcome of the process of appraisal of the situation to which the child and parents are exposed. Prior to this, the personal concerns of children and parents are defined and it is pointed out how these can be threatened by the child's disease. We also pay attention to the development of the child's cognitions about emotion, the development of the concept of death in children, and the awareness of one's own death and fear of death in children with cancer.

3.2. The threat to personal concerns

Emotions arise because an event or a situation is relevant to the concerns of a person (Frijda, 1986). In the case of cancer in a child, there is a great threat to the personal concerns of the child and the parents. For the child there is the threat to physical integrity, safety, security, and, above all, threat to loss of life. The child is confronted with strongly aversive events such as pain and intense physical illness resulting from the disease and the treatment. For a shorter or longer period the child is hindered in his or her activities and cannot participate in all the fun and games, like other children do. For the parents there is the threat of losing their child. A child represents a great personal concern for parents. In a study on the motivation to become a parent, Out and Zegveld (1977) identified the following clusters: a child is seen as an important object of care and love; a child gives meaning to life and thus contributes to the parent's identity; a child represents vitality; confirms the relationship between the partners; is the object of personal goals (through the child, the parents can achieve goals which they have never attained themselves); a child is the focus for identification with the larger whole of nature or creation and contributes to the link with society. The degree to which these aspects form a part of the personal concern of the parents determines what is at stake when cancer is diagnosed in their child.

3.3. The development of the child's cognitions about emotion

A complete description of the processes of emotional development in children is not intended here. We will restrict ourselves to those properties of the emotional development which are important for our study and for research methods directed at the emotional reactions of children. The cognitive understanding of emotions is developed reasonably well in 3 to 4 year old children. They are familiar with the basic emotions such as joy, fear, anger, and grief, and understand the relationship between certain events and the emotional reactions which these events evoke. More complex emotions such as shame, pride, and jealousy, being the result of several components of the situation, are not understood until the later developmental stages (10 - 13 years) which, however, does not have to mean that younger children cannot experience these emotions (see Harter, 1979). During the child's development, a distinct shift can be seen in the concept of emotion. A study by Harris et al. (1981) demonstrates, for example, that for younger children (6 years) an emotion consists of two components: a certain event, on the one hand, and the physical reactions and the behavior which this event evokes, on the other hand. Older children (11 years) include a third component, namely the mental state of a person. Between the fifth and tenth year, children show a progressively greater ability to comprehend that the meaning of a situation can be ambivalent and could therefore evoke conflicting emotions (Harter, 1979; Reissland, 1985).

Recognition of emotions in other persons is already present at a very early age. A child of 9 months recognizes the emotions of others (attachment figures) and reacts to the meaning of specific expressions of emotion. Moreover, at this early age the child already understands that the emotional expression of others contains information about the environment. In unfamiliar situations, the child attempts to come to an appraisal by screening the emotional signals (vocal and facial expressions) of, for instance, the mother (see Bretherton et al., 1986). Another aspect of the recognition of emotions has to do with the recognition of genuine and simulated emotions in others. The child is already capable of this at a very early age. Cummings et al. (1981) found that one to two year old children can already make a distinction between genuine and faked emotions. Saarni (1979) and Harris et al. (1981) demonstrated that six year olds are not only aware that emotions can be simulated, but also that people do not always express their emotions, or that an emotion can be expressed which is different from the emotion that is actually felt. In this respect, it is interesting to raise the point about what children rely on when they are confronted with another person's emotion which does not correspond to the situation in which the other person is in. You would expect that as the child gets older, it would rely more on the situation than on the emotional expressions of others because the child has learned to understand that emotions can be misleading and can be hidden. However, this cannot be clearly proven (see Wiggers, 1984). Some have indeed found that older children do rely more on the situation. But, on the contrary, others have found that it is the younger child who relies more on the situation, and yet another group of researchers has found no difference at all between younger and older children.

The ability to communicate verbally about emotions increases considerably from the second year onwards (see Bretherton et al., 1986). The vocabulary for naming emotions develops quickly. The child uses emotion words to comment on its own and other person's emotions and to explain them, the child can discuss the causes and effects of emotions, and can refer to emotions from the past (reflection) and in the future (anticipation). Bretherton et al. (1986) point out that verbal reflection on emotions often occur in the context of emotion-arousing events which, according to them, illustrates that the ability to discuss

28   *Children with Cancer*

emotions has an important regulatory and clarifying function for the child's interpersonal relationships, even for very young children.

From the above, we can conclude that, even in very young children, emotional reactions can be determined by their verbal expressions. To a certain extent, young children possess the ability to reflect on their own emotional behavior and that of others, and are already capable of linking emotional reactions to emotion-arousing events.

3.4. The development of the death concept in children

Only a limited number of empirical studies has been conducted on what the notion of death means to a child and how this concept changes during the child's development. From this research it emerges that the death concept of a child bears a certain relationship with the age and level of development, but is certainly not entirely determined by these factors. Understanding death as universal and final is generally not found among 3 to 5 year olds (Childers & Wimmer, 1971; Gartley & Bernasconi, 1967; Hansen, 1973; Nagy, 1948; Swain, 1976; White et al., 1978). In this age group children usually see death as a temporary separation or sleep which does not happen to everyone and which can be reversed. The pre-operational developmental stage which these children are in is characterized by egocentricity (the children can only see the world from their own perspective), by animism, magical thinking, and fantasy reasoning (Piaget & Inhelder, 1969). Thinking about death is a reflection of this cognitive developmental stage. However, the stage of cognitive development does not appear to be the major determining factor because Beauchamps (1974) proved that a rather large group of 5 year old children already understood the universality and finality of death and were realistic about causes of death. Most of the other researchers demonstrated that comprehending the finality of death is not present until the age of 7 or 8, and understanding the universality of death develops abruptly at this age (Childers & Wimmer, 1971; White et al., 1978). Between children in the concrete-operational developmental stage (from about 7 to 11 years) and children in the formal-operational developmental stage (from about 12 years), hardly any differences are encountered as to their death concept (Koocher, 1973). The awareness of personal mortality and finality does not exclude the fact that children, just like adults, often use an escape clause, whether based on religious belief or not, of an eternal life or a return to earth by way of reincarnation.

The aforementioned empirical research into the death concept of children was exclusively conducted among healthy children. Not one of the studies examined whether personal experiences with death influenced the development of the death concept. Whether having a life-threatening disease speeds up the development of the death concept of children has not been empirically examined, as far as we know.

3.5. Awareness of one's own death and fear of death of children with cancer

It has often been speculated upon whether a seriously ill child can be aware of impending death and can experience fear of death. Up to the '70's when childhood cancer almost always had a fatal outcome, it was generally accepted that children under ten years could not be aware of their impending death and could therefore not experience fear of death, because their death concept up to that age would be insufficiently developed. In many descriptions of children with cancer it was postulated that death - as an unavoidable and irreversible physiological process - is an abstract concept that only means something to a child who possesses the ability of abstract thought. Attaining the formal-operational developmental stage would be a prerequisite for this. According to various authors (Green, 1967; Natterson & Knudson, 1960; Schowalter, 1970), their clinical impressions of fatally ill children confirmed this assumption. Among children up to about the age of 6 they mainly observed a strong fear of separation, and among children from 6 to 10 years they mainly observed a fear of damage to and mutilation of their body. They did not notice an actual fear of death until the children were older than 10 years. We find it hard to avoid the impression that the clinical observations of these authors are highly influenced by excessive generalizations about the development of the child's thought processes and mainly gratify their own desires. After all, the death of a child is a very emotional experience. It is a comforting thought for adults that the impending death can be hidden from the child, that the child will not be aware of this, and will not experience fear.

Systematic observations of children who died in hospital have caused doubt concerning the tenability of the assumption that children under 10 years of age are not aware of their impending death. Bluebond-Langner (1975, 1977) observed children with leukemia and noticed that all children, even children under 3 years, were aware that they were going to die before the dying stage had actually been reached. This awareness occurred in spite of the fact that parents and hospital staff held back information on the seriousness of the disease and the impending death. According to Bluebond-Langner, as a result of the deterioration of their condition and the emotions and tension around them, the children became aware that they were going to die. She inferred this from a cluster of different types of behavior, sporadic disclosures, and death themes in play and drawings of the children. The awareness process entails several stages, according to the author. From the moment that the diagnosis has been made, the child is aware that the disease is serious but is confident that treatment will lead to a cure. However, when the treatment does not appear to be successful, awareness that one is ill but will be cured shifts to awareness that one will always be ill and will never get better. It is not until the final stage that the child becomes aware that he or she will die. But this stage has already been reached before the dying stage of the child actually sets in. Bluebond-Langner noted that experiences with the death of fellow patients only influenced the awareness process if the child had had a number of relapses. Not until then does the child come to the conclusion that he or she is also going to die.

Glaser and Strauss (1965) use the term awareness context for describing the awareness of impending death, the behavior of a terminal patient, and especially the interactions with relatives and hospital staff. They distinguish four types of awareness contexts: closed awareness, suspected awareness, mutual pretense awareness, and open awareness. In the closed awareness context, a patient is not aware of impending death, and other persons around the patient attempt to prevent the patient becoming aware of this. By the remarks and behavior of others and by events in the environment, the patient can begin to suspect and try to gain confirmation or refutation. If the environment, intentionally or unintentionally, confirms the patient's suspicions, and the patient perceives this as such, a transition occurs to either the mutual pretense or the open awareness context. In the first case the patient is aware of impending death but acts just like the others, as if nothing is wrong. In the open awareness context the impending death is openly recognized and both the patient and the other persons act according to this prospect. Weisman (1972) uses the term 'middle knowledge' for patients who create the impression that 'they don't know anything', while at a certain level of awareness they have a vague realization of their impending death.

A shift to successive awareness contexts was also observed in children by Bluebond-Langner. As soon as the children realized they were going to die, the interactions between the children and those around them almost always took place within the context of mutual pretense. An open awareness context was very exceptional.

As far as we know, in studies on children with cancer it has never been directly asked, for ethical reasons, whether or to what degree the children experience a fear of death. But Koocher and O'-Malley (1981) measured fear of death with a questionnaire in a group of former young cancer patients who had survived their illness for a long period (an average of 12 years). The cancer patients did not report a greater fear of death than a matched control group of patients with a chronic but non-life-threatening illness. They also did not differ from population norms.

Among young children (between 6 and 10 years) with leukemia who were kept in the dark as to the nature and seriousness of their illness, Waechter (1971) and Spinetta et al. (1973) found clearly heightened levels of anxiety. Using a projective test and an anxiety questionnaire, Waechter demonstrated that children with leukemia, between the ages of 6 and 10, were more preoccupied with death and experienced more anxiety than children with a chronic but non-life-threatening disease. Spinetta et al. have also demonstrated that children with leukemia, between the ages of 6 and 10, were more concerned about their physical integrity and physical functioning and experienced more anxiety than children with a chronic but non-life-threatening illness. Because the degree of anxiety is so clearly related to the nature of the prognosis, whether or not this anxiety is labelled as death anxiety is more a problem of semantics than of facts, according to Spinetta (1974).

3.6. The situational meaning structure and the emotional reactions of the child

Responsibility for the situation

The need for finding a cause for the disease and to hold someone or something responsible for the misery arising from the disease is certainly also present in children. From a review of the literature by Peters (1978) in which a number of studies on sick children are discussed, it can be concluded that many children hold themselves responsible for their illness and consider their illness to be a punishment for their own deeds, misbehavior, or breaking rules laid down by their parents. It is often assumed that the tendency to blame oneself for the disease decreases as the child becomes older, because a child then has a better understanding of the cause of diseases. However, in a group of hospitalized children from 2 to 14 years, Gips (1956) found that the older children were actually more inclined to blame themselves and to consider their own actions as the cause of the disease.

The medical treatment and procedures are also seen as a kind of punishment by many children. Eiser (1984) discusses a number of studies from which it appears that this view is especially prevalent among younger children. Brewster (1982) found that chronically ill children between the ages of 6 and 8 considered their treatment as a punishment and experienced the medical staff as punishing. At the age of 8, Brewster found a better understanding of the reasons for and the purpose of treatment, but it was not until the age of 11 that children began to see the medical staff as empathic and no longer as punishing. From this it appears that the children hold the doctors and nurses responsible for the pain and discomforts inflicted upon them. It is our experience, however, that children do not often dare to express feelings of anger, evoked by this attribution of responsibility, toward these persons. Because of fear that they will have to endure even more, they express their anger more often towards persons whom they feel are safer. Often these are the parents.

The anger expressed by the child towards the parents is not only a displacement of anger caused by other persons. Many studies have proven that especially young children between 6 months and 4 years of age demonstrate emotional disturbances during hospitalization and for some time afterwards (see Bowlby, 1973; Rutter, 1972; Vernon et al., 1965). These reactions are mostly considered to be related to the separation and the fear of losing attachment figures. For the young child the separation is the same as an intentional abandonment by the parents. Besides this, the parents are now allowing strangers in the hospital to inflict pain, while they had previously always protected the child from danger and pain. Children who consider themselves rejected in this way by parents and feel let down do not only experience fear, but also strong feelings of anger. They express these feelings as reproach and as an effort to make their parents change their behavior (Bowlby, 1973).

Data in the literature on feelings of guilt and anger in chronically ill children and children with cancer are usually based on clinical impressions (Brunnquell & Hall, 1982; Mattson, 1972). An exception to this is the study by Kashani and Hakami (1982). From a standardized psychiatric interview administered to American children with cancer between the ages of 6 and 17, and to their parents, it became apparent that in half of the children anger and irritation occurred relatively often, even in children who had survived their illness for many years. Our own clinical impressions indicate that adolescents with cancer, besides feelings of guilt arising from the conviction that they are responsible for the disease, also have feelings of guilt about the grief and difficulties which they are causing their parents because of the illness (Van Veldhuizen, 1985). Zeltzer et al. (1980) found that adolescents with cancer more often indicate that their disease causes a disruption in their family than adolescents with another chronic illness.

Children who consider themselves jointly responsible for the success of their treatment experience feelings of pride if this result is achieved. An appraisal of joint responsibility is often encouraged. The child is told by doctors and parents that the success of therapy depends on the fighting spirit demonstrated by the child for enduring the aversive and difficult treatment. The positive effect of an appraisal of joint responsibility is that the child does not have to feel like a helpless victim and can be proud if the illness is overcome by a courageous, fighting spirit. The other side of this story is that feelings of guilt arise if the treatment is unsuccessful and the child partly blames him or herself.

Uncontrollability of the situation

The situation in which the child with cancer finds itself is in many ways uncontrollable or only controllable in a limited sense, and is therefore a source of feelings of anxiety, helplessness, and depression. Illness and hospitalization are generally considered to be a primary situation affecting the sense of control of one's own situation and one's own life. To achieve security and control of the situation, the child is highly dependent on the parents or other trusted persons. They create a buffer between the child and the stressful events which the child is exposed to (Susman et al., 1980). Hospitalization results in strong separation anxiety in the young child who, after a stage of violent protest, reverts to apathy, depression, and regressive behavior if separation from the parents is complete and long-lasting (Bowlby, 1973). With respect to children with cancer, it appears that separation anxiety does not only occur among young children, nor does this anxiety only manifest itself during hospitalization. Lansky and Gendel (1978) observed extreme separation anxiety for both children and mothers in about 3% of a population of children with cancer. The children were between 3 and 15 years old, and half of the children were older than 10 years. According to the authors, separation anxiety resulted in a symbiotic mother-child relationship in which the child demonstrated highly regressive behavior. In the home situation the separation anxiety did not diminish and many children developed school phobia. In the previously mentioned study by Kashani and Hakami (1982), separation anxiety was found among 34% of the 6 to 17 year old children with cancer. The same degree of anxiety was found in pre-adolescents and adolescents, while the time interval since the children's diagnosis varied from 1 month to 10 years. In the same study, it appeared that symptoms of depression occurred more often among children with cancer than what was to be expected on the basis of population norms.

The medical treatment and procedures, including bone marrow aspirations, lumbar punctures, and intravenously administered cytostatics, besides causing acute pain, nausea, vomiting, and severe physical discomfort, also cause acute anxiety. Using systematic behavioral observations, Katz et al. (1980) found that almost all children displayed anxiety and nervous behavior during a bone marrow aspiration. In successive procedures, no habituation seemed to occur in the children. The same observation was made by Van Aken et al. (1986). Conditioned anticipation anxiety and anticipatory nausea and vomiting is a fairly frequent reaction of children to repeated medical procedures and the administering of cytostatics (Dolgin et al., 1985; Katz et al., 1980; Michael & Copeland, 1985). Various therapeutic interventions are applied to give the children some control over their situation and to diminish anxiety, pain, nausea, and vomiting (Van Aken et al., 1986; Dash, 1980; Hilgard & LeBaron, 1982; Kellerman et al., 1983; Zeltzer et al., 1983; Zeltzer & LeBaron, 1982). Adolescents with cancer say treatment is worse than the disease itself and have more problems concerning the treatment than peers with other chronic or serious illnesses (Zeltzer et al., 1980). Spinetta and Maloney (1975) found that 6 to 10 year old children with leukemia undergoing outpatient treatment, experience more anxiety during their visits to the clinic as the disease progresses and with each visit to the clinic.

Treatment of cancer is associated with a number of temporary or permanent physical changes such as baldness, severe weight loss or weight gain, and sometimes deformities as a result of operations. It is assumed that this physical change has a negative influence on the child and especially the adolescent regarding body image, self-confidence, self-esteem, contacts with peers, and school attendance (Kagen-Goodheart, 1977). However for adolescents with cancer, Kellerman et al. (1980) could not find any influence on self-esteem. The adolescents did not differ from peers with other chronic or serious illnesses, nor from healthy peers in their self-esteem. In the same study, Zeltzer et al. (1980) did prove that adolescents with cancer, when compared to healthy peers, did have a more distorted body image and did report more problems at school. All adolescents showed more anxiety, less positive self-esteem, and less control over their disease, if they experienced the impact of the disease on their daily lives as more disruptive. Lansky et al. (1975) pointed out that quite a few children with cancer develop school phobia during their illness. Their observation could not be confirmed by other researchers, although absence from school frequently occurs among many of the children (Deasy-Spinetta, 1981; Eiser, 1980; Henning & Fritz, 1983; Last et al., 1982a). Deasy-Spinetta (1981) studied children in the school situation and demonstrated that children with cancer, compared to their classmates, displayed more withdrawal and timidity and played a more passive role in social contacts. These findings were confirmed in a replication study conducted in the Emma Kinder Ziekenhuis (Blom et al., 1984). In a number of other studies as well, a significant degree of withdrawal was found in children with cancer (Kashani & Hakami, 1982; Last et al., 1982a).

Kellerman et al. (1980) did a study on the 'locus of control' of healthy and chronically ill adolescents. This concerns the confidence that adolescents have in their ability to exercise influence over their own lives and their own future. Adolescents with cancer appeared to attribute less control to themselves in comparison with healthy peers. They saw their life and future mainly determined by fate and other external circumstances. Nannis et al. (1982) interviewed adolescents with cancer (12 to 20 years) who had a poor prognosis. From this study it clearly emerged that these adolescents use some type of illusory control (see section 2.3). Most adolescents were far more optimistic and hopeful about their future than their physical condition allowed. The adolescents had detailed plans for the future which, as the authors indicated, would be considered unrealistic by outsiders. This coping style enables the adolescents to maintain a sense of control over the situation and reduces feelings of helplessness.

Uncertainty about the situation

The unpredictability of the course of the illness and the prolonged uncertainty about the final outcome are the most distinguishing characteristics of cancer. Hope and fear are the emotions which result from uncertainty about future events. In the previously mentioned study by Nannis et al. (1982), it appeared that adolescents with cancer were still hopeful about their future, in spite of a poor prognosis. Susman et al. (1982) studied the same group, and reported that during the interview only a few adolescents mentioned the possibility of dying, in spite of the fact that they had been fully informed by their doctor about the disease and the statistical probability of the effectiveness of their treatment. Sinnema (1984) studied a group of Dutch adolescents with cystic fibrosis. Cystic fibrosis is a chronic disorder with a progressive and, in most cases, fatal outcome. The average life expectancy for these patients lies between 16 and 19 years. In the interview, only 5% of the adolescents brought up the topic of the shortened life expectancy and most of them had optimistic expectations for the future. The findings of Kellerman et al. (1980) and Zeltzer et al. (1980) also indicate that most adolescents with cancer have a hopeful attitude towards the future and do not exhibit much fear of a fatal outcome of their disease. The adolescents with cancer did not appear to be more anxious than healthy peers or peers with other diseases. The authors assume that most of the adolescents use a coping style of denial, thereby reinforcing their hope.

In an attempt to study the effect of long-term uncertainty about the final outcome of the disease, Koocher and O'Malley (1981) studied a large group of pediatric cancer survivors. The average age of this group was 18 years (range of 5-37 years) and they had survived the disease by at least 5 years (an average of 12 years). All patients were free of disease symptoms and were not being treated anymore. With respect to their emotional adjustment (measured with a standardized psychiatric interview, a clinical evaluation of the mental state, projective tests, and an evaluation of social contact skills) and their anxiety, depression, and fear of death (measured by questionnaires), the patients did not differ in any way from the general population norms. A small group of cancer patients was compared to a matched control group of patients with a chronic, but non-life-threatening disease. Compared to this group, the cancer patients did show greater adjustment problems, but did not report stronger anxiety, depression, or fear of death. Only 10% indicated they sometimes thought about a recurrence of the disease, and almost all patients used coping styles such as denial, intellectualization, rationalization, and avoidance during the interview. Empirical data on anxiety and preoccupation with death in younger children, as discussed in section 3.5, seem to deviate from the findings among adolescents. Waechter (1971) and Spinetta et al. (1973) suggest a distinct relationship between anxiety and the life-threatening character of the disease. However, the children were studied in the hospital during a period of treatment. These conditions complicate an accurate identification of the source of anxiety for these children.

In the situation of the child with cancer, there are more conditions present which create uncertainty. For example, there is uncertainty about the reactions of the social environment to the disease and to the changes in appearance. Henning and Fritz (1983) demonstrated that quite a large number of children (14%) from the patient population required professional support when returning to school after the first period of treatment. Most children anticipated negative reactions from their classmates. They were afraid they would be teased about their changed appearance and were afraid of difficulties when discussing the disease.

Restriction of life-style

Children who frequently stay in hospital are exposed to prolonged restriction of their freedom of movement. During the period of recovery from an operation or during the cycle of chemotherapy, freedom of movement is minimal. This situation leads to feelings of anger and frustration. Yet it is remarkable that these feelings are seldom described in the literature on children with cancer. Rather the descriptions found are of passive, quiet, and resigned behavior (Richmond & Waisman, 1955). Susman et al. (1981) conducted a systematic behavioral observation of children who were undergoing a cycle of chemotherapy and came to the conclusion that the passive behavior and withdrawal demonstrated by a fairly large number of children could not be entirely attributed to the toxicity of the drugs. This behavior continued after finishing the cycle of chemotherapy and after the physical condition of the child had improved. For a number of children, the passive behavior and withdrawal seemed to be an indication of depression. In this section, a number of studies were already discussed which showed that withdrawal and a passive and wait-and-see attitude in social contacts were also characteristic of children with cancer who were not hospitalized. In only one case researchers reported, besides withdrawal and quiet behavior, many expressions of anger and frustration in the children (Kashani & Hakami, 1982).

The restriction of the child's life-style due to frequent hospitalization and physical restraints as a consequence of the disease and/or the treatment, results directly or indirectly in social isolation. If the child is often in hospital and does not regularly attend school, the continuity of friendships is broken and social contacts are lost. This social isolation leads to feelings of loneliness. Spinetta and Maloney (1975) found that children with cancer experience more feelings of loneliness than other chronically ill children. Krulik (1978) demonstrated that children with cancer and children with cystic fibrosis are more socially isolated and experience more feelings of loneliness than healthy peers. The social isolation is enhanced because children begin to feel alienated from their peers, do not share their experiences with them anymore, and keep their feelings to themselves (Blom et al., 1984; Deasy-Spinetta, 1981). Social isolation was also demonstrated among adolescents. Sinnema (1984) found that adolescents with cystic fibrosis participated less often in social activities outside the home than adolescents with asthma and healthy adolescents. Adolescents with cancer also reported relatively often that, due to their illness, they had to give up activities outside the home (sports, club membership) and had to spend more time at home (Last et al., 1979).

3.7. The situational meaning structure and the emotional reactions of the parents

Responsibility for the situation

Empirical research directed at the question to what extent parents of children with cancer hold someone or something responsible for their child's illness is limited to a few descriptive studies. On the basis of discussions with parents in the hospital, Bozeman et al. (1955), Friedman et al. (1963), and Chodoff et al. (1964) concluded that many parents feel guilty about the child's illness. In a study involving a large number of parents, it appeared that many parents spontaneously mentioned that they discussed with their spouse and with the doctor whether they could have caused their child's illness (Koocher & O'Malley, 1981). However, none of these studies systematically investigated parental feelings of guilt. On the basis of our own clinical impressions, we assume that parents do experience guilt feelings. These feelings are based on doubts whether they have responded quickly enough to the child's complaints and whether the (family) doctor had referred the child to a pediatrician in time. Parents do not only feel guilty about this but are often angry as well. In a study on home care for families with a child who has cancer, it was found that parents had considerably less appreciation for the family doctor than for the district nurse (Last et al., 1982b). This phenomenon may be partly explained by the parents' need to hold someone responsible and blame someone for the situation. In the descriptive study by Bozeman et al. (1955), it was observed that parents directed their anger at the doctor who told them the diagnosis. Friedman et al. (1963) observed that parents of children with cancer directed their anger towards the pediatrician if the child's condition deteriorates and the child is expected to die. The doctor on whom all hope had been focused is held responsible for that situation. From discussions with parents who participated in considering different treatment options for their child, it appears that this responsibility can weigh very heavily on them. The parents may feel guilty about a possible 'wrong' choice which they have made (Adams, 1978; Last, 1985).

In various studies of parents with chronically ill children, it has been ascertained that the pedagogical relationship changes and the parents adopt a strongly protective attitude towards the sick child. This is found among parents of children with cystic fibrosis (Burton, 1975), with epilepsy (Suurmeyer, 1980), with mental handicaps (Gresnigt & Gresnigt-Strengers, 1973), with asthma (Parker & Lipscombe, 1979), and among parents of seriously ill and dying children (Bonekamp, 1980). A change in child-rearing style, characterized by both over-protection and indulgence, is also described among parents of children with cancer (Adams, 1978; Binger et al., 1969; Fife, 1978). As far as we know, objective research into changes in child-rearing style among parents of children with cancer has not been conducted. The shift in parental attitude towards more protection of the child can be explained, among other things, by the responsibility which the parents feel for the physical condition of the child, which commonly deteriorates due to disease and treatment. It can also be seen as a reaction to the fear of losing the child. An attitude of greater indulgence towards the sick child can be the result of feelings of guilt. The parents may feel guilty because they have been unable to protect their child from the distressing situation which the child is being exposed to. The uncertainty of expectations for the future also plays a role here. After all, raising children is an activity directed towards future goals. The point of making demands of a child in order to achieve goals of upbringing is no longer obvious if there is considerable doubt about the child having a future (Bonekamp, 1980). In a few small-scale studies (Cairns et al., 1979; Kramer, 1984), an attention shift in the family from the other children to the sick child has been demonstrated. Our own clinical impressions suggest that many parents are aware of this attention shift and feel guilty towards their other children. They feel they are neglecting them.

Uncontrollability of the situation

The influence parents can exercise on the disease process is very limited. The potential control created by treatment mostly lies in the hands of the doctor. Moreover, during hospital stays the parents must entrust an important part of the care for the child to others. In descriptive studies of parents of children with cancer, feelings of helplessness are often mentioned (Friedman et al., 1963; Knudson & Natterson, 1960). In an attempt to reduce the experienced uncontrollability, many parents search for a reason why it had to be their child who has been stricken with the disease. This can motivate them to actively gather information on the disease (Friedman, et al., 1963; Koocher & O'Malley, 1981). Empirical research among parents of children with cancer has demonstrated psychological stress reactions, including increased levels of anxiety and depression (Magni et al., 1983; Maguire, 1983; Powazek et al., 1980). In Maguire's (1983) longitudinal study on 60 mothers of children with leukemia, higher levels of anxiety were found in 30% of the mothers shortly after diagnosis and in 25% of the mothers one year later. Depression symptoms were found in 28% of the mothers. These reactions were observed to a much lesser degree in a control group of parents whose children had a non-life-threatening disease. A study by Magni et al. (1983) on a small number of parents of children with leukemia showed significantly higher levels of anxiety and depression in both mothers and fathers shortly after diagnosis, than in a control group matched for age, sex, and socio-economic status. In a retest eight months later, these differences were still present.

In addition to psychological stress reactions, somatic stress reactions were also observed in parents. In a study on a small group of parents of children with leukemia, Powazek et al. (1980) found increased psychosomatic complaints in 88% of the parents in the first half year after diagnosis. In the study by Magni et al. (1983), significantly more sleep disorders were observed in parents of children with leukemia than in the control group, both shortly after diagnosis and eight months later. In her study on the parents of 22 children with cancer, Márky (1982) found that 50% of the mothers and 33% of the fathers did not feel quite healthy during the treatment of their child. The duration of the treatment varied between 3 and 23 months. In the follow-up one year later, 40% of the mothers and 13% of the fathers still reported psychosomatic complaints. They often had to think about their child's illness, felt tired, and often had headaches. They attributed the complaints to the situation and for this reason did not visit their family doctor more often than in the past.

Uncertainty about the situation

Due to improved treatment methods, certainties and uncertainties of the situation for parents of children with cancer have changed considerably in the last decades. In early publications on the emotional reactions of parents of children with cancer, descriptions focus on reactions of parents confronted with a certain, unavoidable loss. The observed reactions of denial, anger, grief, despair, and finally acceptance of the loss (Binger et al., 1969; Chodoff et al., 1964; Friedman et al., 1963; Knapp & Hansen, 1973), demonstrate similarities to findings among persons going through a mourning process after the death of a loved one (Parkes, 1972) and to reactions observed among terminal patients (Kübler-Ross, 1969). The concept of anticipatory grief is used to describe these reactions. Mourning over a loss which has not yet occurred constitutes the unique character of anticipatory grief (Weisman, 1974). Reactions of anticipatory grief arise due to the expectation that loss is certain. In the light of a certain fatal outcome of the disease process, reactions of anticipatory grief are described as part of an adequate adjustment to the situation created by the disease (Friedman, 1967; Futterman & Hoffman, 1973; Townes et al., 1974). An advanced process of anticipatory grief has implications for the relationship with the person whom one is expecting to lose. An affective alienation develops gradually. This phenomenon was first described by Lindemann (1944) among women whose soldier husbands served at the European front, but against all their expectations these husbands survived. If a parent resigns him or herself to losing the child but the child survives contrary to expectations, this can result in the parent being unable to maintain an emotional bond with the child. In a study on behavioral disorders of children who survived contrary to expectations, Green and Solnit (1964) call this the 'vulnerable child syndrome'. The behavioral disorders are the result of a permanently disrupted parent-child relationship. In some cases this syndrome is also observed in children with cancer (Koocher & O'Malley, 1981). Modern cancer treatment has resulted in making the outcome of the disease uncertain. Depending on the circumstances, parents go through many mood changes. In a study of parents who participated in a discussion group for parents of children with cancer, it was observed that feelings of fear and tension increased if the child was readmitted to hospital for tests or treatment, if a relapse or recurrence occurred, or if complications arose due to the treatment. Feelings of hope and confidence increased if remission was achieved and if test results were favorable (De Geus & Last, 1983).

In addition to the distress which parents experience in connection with the treatment of their own child, experiences with fellow patients can also be an important source of uncertainty. One of the most overwhelming experiences is the death of another child with cancer. In a study by Kalnins et al. (1980), it was demonstrated that in 35% of the families of children with leukemia, family members became very disturbed when another child suffering from leukemia died. Interviews with the parents showed that their fear of a fatal outcome of the disease for their own child was strongly enhanced by this experience. The long duration of the disease, especially if the child's condition deteriorates, may evoke fear in parents that they will not be able to endure it any longer. Many parents who lost a child with leukemia described this fear in interviews when talking about the long days beside the sickbed in the final stage before their child's death (Lascari & Stehbens, 1973). Even if the child's illness takes a favorable course, it does not mean that parents are entirely freed from the fear of a recurrence of the disease. In the study by Koocher and O'Malley (1981), it was found that fear of a recurrence of their child's disease remained in the parents' mind, in spite of the number of years that had passed. The children of these parents had survived their illness by an average of 12 years. Many parents said they were overly sensitive to disease symptoms which had initially appeared in their child.

Restriction of life-style

During hospitalization, parents spend much time with their sick child. But even after the period of hospitalization normal habits must be adjusted to the changed situation. The restrictions associated with the illness can be a source of frustration, anger, feelings of loneliness, and of isolation from the social environment for the parents. In a few studies it was found that parents who had professional jobs outside the home experienced this, on the one hand, as a kind of distraction (Márky, 1982). On the other hand, the job situation can become a source of stress because the parents thoughts are with the child and thus they may feel they are not functioning as well as they should (Cook, 1984; Koocher & O'Malley, 1981).

Many other sources of stress in the family, directly or indirectly related to the child's illness, can increase the parents' feelings of being restricted in life-style. Research into this subject provides evidence indicating that besides problems at work, problems with the other children, financial problems, and relational problems also exist (Kalnins et al., 1980; Kreuger et al., 1981; Kupst & Schulman, 1980). In the longitudinal study by Kalnins et al. (1980), the existence of one or more of these problems was ascertained in 44% of the families. The extra costs incurred by the illness may also contribute to restriction of freedom which the parents experience. In American studies it was found that more than 30% of the weekly family budget was spent on medical and non-medical treatment-related expenses (Lansky et al., 1979, 1983).

The child's illness can also influence the feeling of being free in the relationship between the parents. In Maguire's (1983) study on mothers of children with leukemia, it was found that 20% of the mothers had not had sexual contact with their partner since their child's diagnosis or did not experience pleasure from it anymore. They felt tense and also guilty if they would be enjoying themselves while their child was so ill. However, various studies indicate that parents support each other considerably. Murstein (1960) found that a good marital relationship is associated with a good emotional adjustment to the situation. Morrow et al. (1984) also found a strong relationship between support from the partner and adjustment to the situation during the child's treatment. This relationship could not be demonstrated if the child is doing well and treatment had been finished. An explanation of this finding could be that parents are very much dependent on each other, especially during the treatment stage, when they have to share tasks and make arrangements for the family. This study though, shows that younger parents (under 30 years) experience more difficulties in adjusting to the situation than older parents. A similar result was found by Kupst et al. (1982). They studied the coping style in parents of children with leukemia, shortly after diagnosis and one year later. Families in which the child was young had more coping problems than families in which the child was older. Yet after one year most of the families seemed to cope adequately with the disease. Adjustment after one year could not be predicted on the basis of the coping behavior shortly after diagnosis. The fluctuations occurring in the parents' adjustment could not be attributed to the course of the child's illness but to additional family problems, including marital and financial problems.

Considering that parents have to make an effort to cope with the situation as best as possible for such a long time, presumably this leads to tensions and even to disruptions in their relationship. From an investigation into the incidence of divorces among parents of children with cancer it was concluded, however, that divorces are not more frequent than in the total population (Kalnins et al., 1980; Lansky et al., 1978). In the study by Lansky et al. (1978), relational problems were observed among parents of children with cancer. They have more relational problems than parents in the 'normal' population, but less than parents who seek counselling therapy because of relational problems. In spite of the marital tension which can arise, many parents feel the situation created by the disease has deepened their relationship. In the study by Koocher and O'Malley (1981), 70% of the parents indicated they had achieved a more strongly-knit bond with their partner and 86% indicated they had grown closer together as parents.

Many parents experience a restriction in their social contacts. In many descriptions it is pointed out that parents of children with cancer do not have the energy anymore to show interest in the day to day worries of others and become irritated by how others expect them to behave. It is also described how others withdraw, finding it difficult to determine what kind of attitude they should adopt and not knowing how to cope with their own anxiety with respect to the disease (Bozeman et al., 1955; Friedman et al., 1963; Heffron et al., 1973; Lansky, 1974). From research into the relationship between sources of support and the parent's adaptation to the situation, however, Morrow et al. (1984) conclude that parents receive substantial support, not only from the spouse, but also from relatives and friends. In the study by Koocher and O'Malley (1981), parents do not really experience emotional support from relatives and friends, but feel more supported by offers of practical help. For many parents a shift in values seems to take place during the disease period. Goals which had previously been considered important, now become less important or not important at all. This re-evaluation can be considered as an intra-psychic defense against the frustrations caused by the restriction of life-style. Many parents experience positive feelings from this changed orientation towards life.

Sex differences in the parents' emotional reactions

In literature on the emotional reactions of the parents of children with cancer, differences in emotional responses between fathers and mothers are regularly reported. These findings are based on clinical impressions and empirical research. In various studies, higher levels of depression are found in mothers than in fathers (Kupst & Schulman, 1980; Magni et al., 1983; Townes et al., 1974). In the study by Magni et al. (1983), fathers scored lower than mothers on all scales of distress. The fathers only scored higher on the anger scale. In her study, Márky (1982) observed that during the child's treatment, mothers show more psychosomatic complaints than fathers. In studies on grief reactions of parents after the death of their child, a higher degree of distress is again found in mothers. The fathers are designated as being inclined to accept the situation more easily (Rando, 1983; Townes et al., 1974).

Differences in emotional reactions between fathers and mothers are often attributed in the literature to the fact that caring for the sick child is usually the mother's task (Koocher & O'Malley, 1981), while fathers continue their work and often find distraction therein (Márky, 1982). On the other hand, it has been demonstrated that fathers of children with cancer often think about their sick child and therefore do not function well in their jobs anymore (Cook, 1984). Cook (1984) points out that the difference in social roles between fathers and mothers often entails differences in problem-orientation. The mothers are more intensely involved with caring for the sick child, while the fathers orient themselves more to tasks which will guarantee the economic continuity of the family. The study by Cook was conducted among a large group of American parents (90 mothers and 55 fathers). Compared to the fathers, the mothers appear to have more problems with communicating about the disease with their child and with motivating the child to accept treatment. They also experience more problems in their marital relationship. Mothers more often feel they cannot keep it up and experience more feelings of helplessness and social isolation. Moreover, they doubt whether they are a good mother. Fathers, on the contrary, have more problems with their jobs and feel more excluded due to the greater involvement of the mother with the sick child.

A difference in task orientation between the parents may influence the appraisal of the situation, resulting in different emotional responses. We must take into account, however, universal differences between men and women in expressing and reporting emotions. Women generally report more physical and psychological stress complaints and less well-being than men (Ormel, 1980b). But this does not mean that they also experience more tension in general. The differences found between fathers and mothers may be based on a difference in inclination to express emotions or to report or deny emotions. In this respect, it is important to mention that none of the studies on the emotional experiences of parents of children with cancer examined the influence of defense mechanisms.

4. Communication about the disease

4.1. The concept of communication

The numerous definitions of the concept of human communication found in the literature can, as stated by Nilsen (1970), be divided into definitions which limit the concept of communication to specific kinds of human interactions and definitions, without any restrictions, which count all kinds of human interaction as communication. The term communication, derived from the Latin word 'communicare' which means to share something with somebody, in everyday language means giving information or exchanging ideas or opinions and so refers to a specific form of human interaction. Also belonging to this category are definitions in the literature in which communication is defined from the perspective of the sender, from the person who generates stimuli with the intention of evoking a response from another person, the receiver (Nilsen, 1970). Moreover, not every transmission of stimuli from one person to another is called communication, but only those stimuli or types of behavior which are transmitted as signs or symbols through verbal or non-verbal channels. Behavior in the form of signs or symbols, also called a code or message, must have a common meaning for individuals within the same culture before it can be counted as communicative behavior (Wiener et al., 1972).

Definitions of communication based on the perspective of the receiver do not distinguish between types of behavior or intentionality of the behavior. For example, Ruesch and Bateson (1951) are of the opinion that all behavior is potentially communicative behavior. When somebody perceives the appearance or the behavior of another person and infers some meaning from it, interprets it, then communication has taken place. In the immediate presence of another person, everything that is done can be meaningful to the other and, given the fact that one cannot not behave, it is equally impossible not to engage in communication in someone else's presence (Watzlawick et al., 1967). In this view, a message is not restricted to behavior in the form of signs or symbols, transmitted through language or non-verbal behavior, such as certain gestures or facial expressions. Neither is it required that the behavior must be part of a socially-shared reference system. Activity and inactivity, words and silences, are all messages if they are perceived and interpreted by another, even if they occur in an entirely idiosyncratic manner. Dance (1967) stipulates that the minimal requirement for communication is a response from the receiver. But this response does not have to be manifest. According to Penman (1980), the requirement of a response can be reduced to the requirement that a receiver of the message must be present. As soon as there is someone to receive the message there is always a response, even if the response consists of silence. When defining communication from the perspective of the receiver, it is not necessary to include the intention of the sender. Whether or not a sender intended anything by the message is not a determinant for the response from the receiver (Nilsen, 1970). The response is influenced by the intentions which the receiver of a message surmises or perceives from the sender. The child with cancer who stays in hospital and observes that a fellow patient is dying, while neither parents nor nurses discuss this with him or her, can suspect the intention behind this silence that they consider him or her to be too young to understand what is happening. The child may respond either by asking questions about this event or by choosing to remain silent.

From this view of communication in which the perception and interpretation of the receiver take a central position, it is only a small step to defining the concept of human communication as the process of appraisal. This step has been taken by Barnlund (1970) and Sereno and Bodaken (1975), among others. Besides interpersonal communication, being the appraisal of stimuli originating from another person, these authors also use the concept of intrapersonal communication. Intrapersonal communication concerns the process of appraisal, the interpretation of each stimulus which is perceived by a person. Thus it is a process which does not require the presence of another person. But the concept of communication is then so broadly defined that it has become identical to the concept of cognition. This does not really get us anywhere. In cognitive approaches to emotion, cognitive processes form an important part of the emotion process, but this does not mean that cognition is identical to emotion. The same applies to communication. Cognitive processes also play an important role here, but it is going too far to say that these processes are identical to communication.

In our opinion, a useful definition of the concept of communication is a definition which includes the perspective of the sender and/or the perspective of the receiver. Communication can then be defined as the process of exchange of information between at least two persons who are in each other's perceptual field.

4.2. The function of communication

Communication established through the exchange of messages between persons has a dual function, according to most authors. On the one hand, communication has the function of transmitting information to another person. On the other hand, it's function is to define, maintain, or alter the relationship with the other person (Penman, 1980). Both functions are performed simultaneously and correspond to what Danziger (1976) calls the functions of presentation and representation. Presentation is related to the informational function of communication, of providing information on events taking place within or around the individual. Representation concerns the relational function of communication. It is the expression of the nature of the relationship existing between persons. By presenting oneself in a certain way, a person defines his or her role in each relationship with others. The doctor-patient relationship and the parent-child relationship are typical examples of relationships where the social roles of the communicating partners are complementary and take shape in communication.

The same distinction between informational and relational functions is made by Watzlawick et al. (1967). In each message they distinguish a report aspect and a command aspect. The report aspect is concerned with the content of the message, conveying information about facts, opinions, beliefs, etc. The command aspect is an implicit or explicit commentary on the way in which the content of the message should be interpreted by the other person. It imposes a certain behavior upon the other person and, as such, defines the relationship between the communicating persons. The command aspect corresponds to the terms purport and intended effect used by Van Heerden (1977). The command aspect is of a higher logical type than the report aspect. The first is actually communication about the communication and is thus metacommunication. In conflicts about the nature of the relationship, the command aspect is more prominent, while the report aspect of communication is less important. The report aspect is more important if the relationship between persons is accepted, but both aspects are present in every message (Watzlawick et al., 1967). The distinction between the functions or aspects of communication may be clarified by an example. The doctor's statement to a child with cancer: "It is a disease which you must fight against" is a statement which refers to the actual situation. The child has a disease which cannot be fought without the efforts of those involved. The purport and the intended effect of this statement is not immediately clear. Is it an assertion, a warning, a request, an order, an encouragement, or a threat? Is the doctor attempting to encourage the child to do his or her best for the treatment? Is the doctor warning the child that the treatment will be hard to bear or is it a menace that the child will not get better if he or she does not show a fighting spirit? Can the child infer from this that it will be his or her own fault if he or she does not get well? How the child interprets the above message depends on the non-verbal behavior accompanying the statement and the context in which the message is given.

The information gained from the situation in which a statement has been made, the non-verbal behavior including vocalizations such as voice pitch, intonation, speed, and pauses, the facial expression, glance, gestures, and posture, and also the status and position of the speaker are all factors which determine the purport of the message. These factors provide the receiver of the message with the orientation necessary for checking whether the intentions of the speaker have been correctly interpreted (Van Heerden, 1977). The speaker may make the intention of the message more explicit: "I am warning you...", but this usually remains implicit. In the literature, the term digital is used for the verbal explicit part of a message and the term analog for the non-verbal implicit part of a message. Penman (1980) also relates these components of a message to a manifest and a latent level on which a message can be analyzed. The following figure shows the model of a message as outlined by Penman.

Here the manifest level concerns the explicit information or the literal content of a message such as in the statement "It is a disease which you must fight against". The latent level also contains all the relevant aspects of the context of a message. The implicit content of the statement "It is a disease which you must fight against", can after all mean for the child, given the context in which the statement is made: "Otherwise you will not get better" or "otherwise you will die". Inconsistencies or contradictions in the entire message may occur within and between all the components and levels. Contradictions or incongruencies between levels are assumed to be most significant in defining the nature of the relationship between persons in general (Haley, 1976).

Figure 4.2.1
A model of the message and levels for its description by Penman (1980).

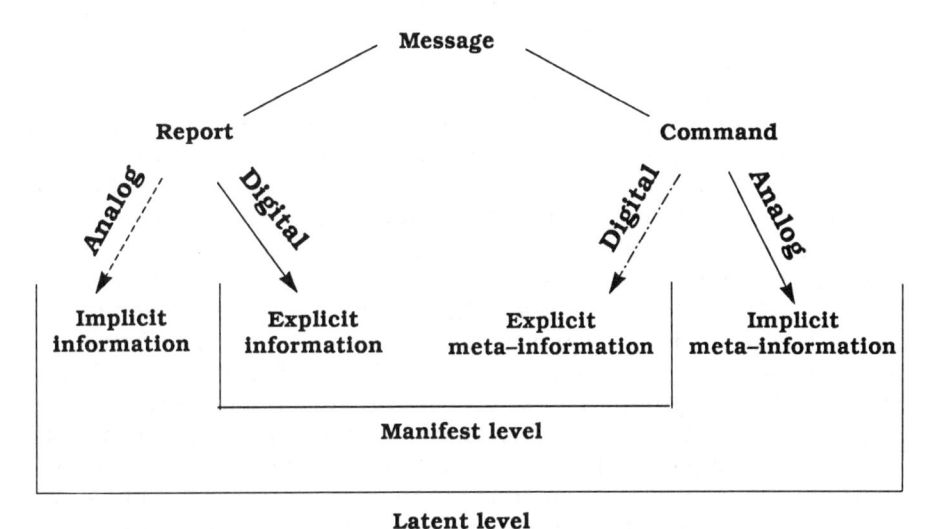

```
                          Message
                         /       \
                  Report           Command
                 /    \             /     \
           Analog   Digital    Digital   Analog
              ↓       ↓           ↓         ↓
         Implicit  Explicit   Explicit   Implicit
        information information meta-information meta-information
                   |_____|
                         Manifest level
         |_____|
                          Latent level
```

The function of information in stressful situations

Information on (potentially) threatening events has two important functions. First, it can increase controllability of the situation. Second, it can reduce uncertainty about the situation. Information increases the controllability of a threatening situation if the individual can infer from it what can be done about the situation, how negative consequences can be avoided or ameliorated by one's own actions. Information reduces uncertainty about a threatening situation if it increases the predictability of the situation, if it contains particulars on the nature and/or the time of occurrence of the impending threat. As previously mentioned, uncontrollability and uncertainty are important components of the situational meaning structure and are conditions for the quality and intensity of emotional behavior, including anxiety, grief, despair, and depression. Although they are distinguishable, controllability and certainty as dimensions of the situation are difficult to separate in reality, and even in experimental laboratory research. Knowing what is going to happen does give some measure of control over the situation. Knowing what to do about a situation, should it arise, reduces feelings of uncertainty and presupposes knowledge of the nature of the situation.

Experimental research into the effects of information on stress reactions. From many laboratory experiments it appears that, in general, people prefer to receive information on an impending threat prior to the event. Literature reviews by Averill (1973) and Seligman (1975) indicate that the subject even desires this information in situations where the danger cannot be avoided by direct action or the consequences of the threat cannot be diminished by direct action. However, studies on the effect of prior information on subsequent stress reactions has yielded equivocal results. In some experiments an intensification of stress reactions has been found; in other experiments a reduction of stress reactions have been observed, and sometimes no difference in stress reactions could be demonstrated between individuals who were informed beforehand and those who were not. There are indications that predictability of an impending threat facilitates long-term adaptation, even if there is a short-term intensification of stress reactions (Averill, 1973; Cohen, 1980; Epstein, 1973; Seligman, 1975). To explain this phenomenon, Seligman (1975) devised the safety-signal hypothesis. This hypothesis states that people (and animals), when threatened with traumatic events, remain in a state of continuous fear, unless a signal is present which provides a reliable prediction of safety. A warning signal (prior information) predicts danger, but absence of this signal predicts safety. When providing a warning signal, a safety signal is simultaneously provided so that the individual can relax in the meantime, knowing there is no immediate danger. Without a warning signal, and thus without a safety signal, the individual remains in a constant state of fear. According to this hypothesis, reduction in stress reactions cannot be attributed to information on the impending threat itself, but to the opportunity this information provides to make a distinction between events which are associated with the danger and those which are not.

Effects of information about medical procedures on stress reactions of patients. Research on hospitalized adult patients indicates that most people prefer to receive prior information on an impending threat, such as medical procedures which they must undergo (Visser, 1982). Another similarity with laboratory experiments is that the studies on the effect of information on patients' stress reactions has yielded equivocal results. Most research has been conducted on surgery patients. In some studies, the information given to the patient prior to surgery had a positive effect on the stress reactions post-surgically. In other studies a negative effect was shown, and in a number of studies no effect was found at all (see Ley, 1977). The discrepant findings may be partly attributed to differences in situational factors (nature of the disease, nature of the surgical procedure, nature of the information provided, time of measuring the stress reactions, etc.), but personal factors especially seem to play an important role.

The tendency to avoid or deny threatening events also influences the manner in which the information about threatening events is dealt with. It is difficult to answer the question whether giving information actually decreases or increases the stress reactions of persons who are inclined towards denial. The studies conducted on this subject show contradictory results (Andrew, 1970; Cohen & Lazarus, 1973; DeLong, 1970; Janis, 1969; also see Lazarus & Folkman, 1984). In various studies, Janis (1969) demonstrated that defensive patients avoid preoperative stress-relevant information and experience strong postoperative stress reactions and anxiety. Janis attributes this to a lack of the necessary 'work of worrying' by these patients. According to him, cognitive anticipation is essential for developing effective coping mechanisms for postoperative pain and stress. Burstein and Meichenbaum (1979) observed the same phenomenon in children. Defensive children showed more avoidance of stress-relevant themes (play) prior to hospitalization, and demonstrated more anxiety after discharge than children who were not defensive. These authors also explain their results as the lack of 'work of worrying' by the defensive children.

In a review of studies on the effects of preparing children who have to undergo medical procedures, Eiser (1984) concludes that the effects on the child's emotional behavior do not extend beyond the situation of the actual procedure. Children who have received information just before the procedure, are less anxious immediately before and during the procedure than children who have had no information, but a long-term effect is not demonstrated during the entire hospitalization period. Research into the effects of information on stress reactions is usually performed among children who stay in hospital for a short time and undergo minor procedures or surgery. This limits generalization. The results are not directly applicable to children with a chronic or life-threatening illness who are subjected to frequent and/or lengthy hospitalization and aversive treatment. Furthermore, the effects of information on stress reactions has almost exclusively been studied during the period of hospitalization, while emotional reactions to hospitalization especially manifest themselves in children in the long term (after hospitalization) (Quinton & Rutter, 1976).

4.3. The function of communication about the disease for the child with cancer and the parents

As previously suggested, a life-threatening disease is a situation in which primary control is limited and, partly due to this, the individual has to rely on secondary types of control (Rothbaum et al., 1982). Neither the child with cancer nor the parents are themselves capable of averting the threat created by the disease by way of direct action. For this reason, control of the situation will be sought, among other things, in processes which enable them to understand and accept the situation. The function and effects of information about their situation which parents and children receive or seek can be analyzed in terms of strengthening or weakening the primary and secondary control processes. In this respect it is important to note that safety signals can be imbedded in the situation of the child with cancer and the parents by providing information about the diagnosis and prognosis. McIntosh (1976) observed that cancer patients who were not informed of their condition, continuously scanned their environment for cues indicating threatening danger. They search for the significance of a remark or attitude of the doctor, the significance of a certain procedure or treatment, and compare their condition and treatment with those of other patients who presumably have the same or a similar disease. If a person has information on the diagnosis and prognosis, this person may be better equipped to assess the significance of signals implicated by events and make a distinction between signals which indicate danger and those which do not. Thus a safety signal can be imbedded within the information that is provided.

In searching for and developing control, communication about the disease is an important device for the child and parents. It serves both the primary control of the situation (problem-focused coping) and the secondary control of the situation (emotion-focused coping). Information exchange about the disease and treatment promotes primary control. It enables those involved to define the problem and make attempts to solve the problem. Communication about the disease directed at secondary control of the situation, promotes understanding and acceptance of the disease and aims to reduce negative emotions and strengthen positive emotions.

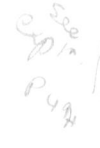

Communication is an important means of appraisal of the situation. The parent who keeps on telling the child it will get better, invites the child to view the situation in a certain (optimistic) way, and thus attempts to reinforce the child's hope and reduce fear. A message is not only intended to change the other's behavior or cognition, but it may also entail an invitation to the other person to alter the cognitions of the person sending the message. The child who has heard of the disease's seriousness may intend by the question "Am I going to die?", that the parents correct the cognition of a fatal outcome of the disease and reassure him or her. It is likely that there is reciprocity between appraisal of the situation and communication about the disease. On the one hand, the function of communication is to develop, maintain, or alter the appraisal; on the other hand, appraisal determines communication. Problems arise in communication if those involved do not share the same appraisal. Van Dantzig (1978) points to this phenomenon in his description of a cancer institute as a 'system of hope'. Communication between patients and hospital staff is obstructed as soon as patients indicate the possibility of a fatal outcome of the disease and express the desire to discuss their fears. Then opportunities for expressing emotions and seeking social support get blocked. The conflict between the need for expressing emotions such as anxiety and grief, on the one hand, and the need for controlling the situation by, for example, avoidance and denial, on the other hand, is solved by communication characterized by symbolic language. An example of this type of communication is provided by a mother who participated in a discussion group for parents of children with cancer. This mother tells about her eleven year old son who talked in his sleep while dreaming. In the morning when she asks which of her children had such troubled sleep, he initially remains silent. She encourages him with: "Was that you? Come on, you can tell your mother everything. Dreams are just lies anyway." Then her son tells her that he had dreamed about a doctor who told him that he should be dead for one year. In the communication between this mother and her son, the expression of fear of death is imbedded in the reassurance that dreams are lies and in the magical conception of a temporary death.

Doctors' opinions on the effects of providing information to the parents of a child with cancer

In the medical literature, highly divergent views can be found on informing the parents of a child with a life-threatening disease. Opinions among doctors range from extreme caution to great frankness. In the Netherlands, especially the pediatrician Veeneklaas (1960, 1962, 1964a, 1964b, 1977) has paid much attention to this topic. He was a definite proponent of the view that one ought to exercise extreme caution when informing the parents of the child's diagnosis and prognosis. In his opinion, knowledge of the course of the illness should be kept from the parents as long as possible. Because terms such as leukemia were already known to the general public through the media in the '60's, he also advised against using terms such as disease of the blood or blood disorders, because their questionable meaning could arouse suspicion. Although withholding information from the parents became more and more difficult due to the parents' increasing awareness, it did not cause Veeneklaas to change his point of view, as is apparent from his publication in 1977. The wish to conceal knowledge about the course of the illness from parents is not only inspired by a certain fatal outcome. Exactly because of the fact that new treatment methods offer the opportunity to cure a number of children with cancer and to extend the children's survival time considerably, De Waal (1973) and Frijling-Schreuder (1973) find it to be too much of a burden for parents to live with the knowledge of the course of the illness longer than a few weeks or months. Frijling-Schreuder points out the danger that parents emotionally withdraw from their child too soon due to a premature mourning process and she indicates the danger of a seriously disturbed parent-child relationship if the child, contrary to expectations, does not die. Moreover, she also objects to lying and secrecy becoming imbedded in the parent-child relationship, with possibly harmful consequences, whenever the fatal prognosis is communicated to the parents but not to the child. Frijling-Schreuder writes:

> "I know it is often said that parents have a right to know as soon as the doctor knows for certain. However, I am personally convinced that whatever the parents know, the child will at least suspect. In this way the secret will become an extra burden in what is already such a problematic relationship between the parents and their seriously ill child" (p. 267).

It should be remarked that each discrepancy between information which the parents have and that which the child receives from the doctor or parents means secrecy in the parent-child relationship. This applies just as much to a possibly fatal prognosis as to a certainly fatal prognosis. Moreover, counteracting the creation of secrecy between parent and child by withholding information from the parents does not mean an actual removal, but is no more than a shift of the problem to the relationship between the doctor and the parents, in which secrecy is just as harmful. Many doctors actually put the emphasis on providing open and honest information about the diagnosis and prognosis, right after the diagnosis has been made, as a necessary condition for establishing a relationship of trust between doctor and parents which is essential during the child's disease process (Ablin et al., 1971; Bakker, 1982; Friedman,

1967; Green, 1967; Greenberg et al., 1984; De Kraker & Voûte, 1973; Kuipers, 1974; Neidhardt & Hertl, 1978; Toch, 1964). Publications and a number of surveys (Novack et al., 1979; Oken, 1961) show that doctors mainly base their attitude towards providing information about a disease such as cancer to patients and family members on their own personal experiences, so it is not surprising that proponents of frankly informing the parents are usually doctors working in specialized cancer centers. Their experiences have convinced them that the truth cannot remain a secret from parents in this environment and that all good intentions to keep secrets, such as presenting the diagnosis as not quite definite or the disease as relatively harmless, are doomed to fail. However, honest and complete information does not imply that doctors always explicitly use the term cancer (Kuipers, 1974). Because of the connotations of this term, the specific medical name of the disease or terms such as tumor or malignant growth are sometimes preferred to the term cancer. Although the taboo associated with the word cancer has lost some of its compulsiveness in the last decades, many doctors and laymen still feel that cancer is a cruel and painful word (Brewin, 1977; McIntosh, 1974). It is also striking that doctors using the word cancer for the sake of complete honesty and openness when discussing the diagnosis, rarely or never use the term in later discussions (Brewin, 1977).

In the United States, legal requirements regarding informed consent have influenced how parents are informed (Greenberg et al., 1984). From a study by Nitschke et al. (1986) among American pediatricians/oncologists, it emerges that all doctors in the initial stage of the disease inform the parents of children with cancer of the diagnosis, prognosis, treatment, and side-effects of treatment. Information on the child's life expectancy in terms of survival rates is given by more than three-quarters of the doctors. In the terminal stage, most doctors (96%) inform the parents on the progression of the child's disease symptoms. However, a large number of doctors (42%) do not talk to the parents about the child's impending death in this stage.

Many doctors make specific recommendations about the manner in which the diagnosis should be presented to the parents and the topics which ought to be discussed then (Ablin et al., 1971; Friedman et al., 1963; Greenberg et al., 1984; Howell, 1966; De Kraker & Voûte, 1973; Kuipers, 1974; Myers, 1983; Neidhardt & Hertl, 1978; Toch, 1964; De Waal, 1973). These recommendations concern the necessity of privacy during the discussion and the importance (if at all possible) of the presence of both parents, in order to prevent that one parent must carry the burden of informing the partner. In this case distortion of the information is unavoidable. Besides transmitting information on the diagnosis, prognosis, treatment plan, and the expected complications, it is considered useful to provide information on the expected reactions of the parents themselves, the sick child, the other family members, and other persons in the environment. An attitude of empathy and understanding of the parents' emotions is considered to be essential. It is also pointed out that it is necessary to repeat information later on in the communication process with the parents because the violent emotions which arise following the news of the diagnosis obstruct the assimilation of information. Strengthening hope by referring to the favorable chances of treatment is thought to be essential. "Clinging to the hope of an effective treatment is the only way for parents to recuperate from the blow caused by learning the diagnosis", according to De Kraker and Voûte (1973). But unjustified optimism is warned against because it may undermine the trust in the doctor (Kuipers, 1974; Pichler et al., 1982). It creates the impression that the doctor does not sufficiently recognize the seriousness of the situation (Green, 1967).

Opinions on the effects of informing the child about the disease

Informing adult cancer patients and children with cancer is more often a topic for discussion than informing next of kin. Not only the medical profession, but social scientists too have joined in this discussion. Brewin (1977) points out that whoever writes about this subject is walking in a minefield and will be classified as belonging either to the school of proponents: those who believe that patients should be told the truth, or to the school of opponents: those who feel that this should not be done. The medical profession is found more often in the school of opponents. Psychiatrists, psychologists, and social workers are more often encountered in the school of proponents: "those who are heavy with words of advice and singularly light in their personal experience", according to Gould and Toghill (1981). It should be noted that the issue 'to tell or not to tell' is almost exclusively associated with cancer patients, even if it concerns adults, and not with diseases having just as serious symptoms and prognoses (Brewin, 1977). Hackett and Weisman (1977) noticed a distinct difference in communication style of doctors and nurses towards cancer patients and towards patients in the acute stage of a serious heart attack. With the former group they were much more hesitant and careful than with the latter, while the survival chances for both groups were comparable. The strong associations of the word cancer with agonizing pain, mutilation, deterioration, destruction, and death are not only present in the layman but also in those who are professionally involved with this disease. Cancer is a metaphor for elusiveness and, literally, malignancy (Sontag, 1979). The opinions on what a child with cancer can be told about his or her disease can be classified into two approaches, according to Share (1972): an open approach and a protective approach. The protective approach consists of protecting the child, as much as possible, from the real meaning of the disease. The environment pretends there is nothing seriously wrong. The open approach consists of informing the child about the diagnosis and prognosis. The life-threatening character of the disease is acknowledged in communication with the child.

Advocates of the protective approach (Evans & Edin, 1968; Frijling-Schreuder, 1973; Howell, 1966; Plank, 1964; Richmond & Waisman, 1955; Toch, 1964; Veeneklaas, 1962, 1977; De Waal, 1973) point out that the child's defense mechanisms are still insufficiently developed to cope with the anxiety aroused by the awareness of the potentially fatal outcome of the disease. Denial and repression of signals pointing to a potentially fatal outcome can only be accomplished if children are supported by adults around them. Another argument for a protective approach is that the child's death concept is still insufficiently developed. By confronting the child with his or her potential death, fearful fantasies associated with the way in which the child views death could arise and be intensified: death as punishment for bad thoughts and deeds, and death as abandonment. As a final justification for a protective approach, it is pointed out that the children themselves tend to remain silent about their illness. From the fact that children often do not ask questions about their illness, it is inferred that the child is presumably not interested in knowledge about the disease. It is assumed that children live from day to day and are more interested in what is actually happening to them, the needle, and the pain experienced at the moment, than in the future. Authors advocating an open approach (Adams-Greenly, 1984; Binger et al., 1969; Bluebond-Langner, 1975, 1977; Issner, 1973; Johnson et al., 1979; Karon, 1973; Karon & Vernick, 1968; Schowalter, 1970; Spinetta, 1978, 1980; Spinetta & Maloney, 1978; Vernick & Karon, 1965; Waechter, 1971; Wolters, 1970) are of the opinion that the facts cannot be kept secret from the child. Withholding information isolates the child from communication which is meaningful in that situation. The child does not feel free to ask questions and to express worries about the disease, so that feelings of loneliness, alienation, and isolation are aroused and intensified. In the authors' opinion, attempts at secrecy are doomed to fail and actually feed the child's unrealistic fearful fantasies. Children will mistrust the adults around them if they discover that they have been misled by them. According to the authors, the child's silence is not a sign that the child is not aware of the seriousness of the disease, but a result of the adults' silence from which the child infers that talking about the disease is not desired or allowed. Karon and Vernick (1968) define this situation as a 'conspiracy of silence'.

Spinetta (1980) makes a case against a number of objections which opponents of open communication put forward. According to him, talking with the child about the diagnosis and prognosis does not mean that the child is told something new. It only gives the child permission to speak freely about his or her worries. According to the author, the child is not better off if his or her suspicions are not confirmed because fear of the unknown - especially for a child - is worse than fear of what is known. If children cannot share their suspicions with others, they become isolated, depressed, and dejected. According to Spinetta, open communication reduces feelings of isolation and despair and promotes positive self-esteem.

Not every publication which discusses informing the child with cancer can be classified according to a strict dichotomy between the open and the protective approach. The pediatricians De Kraker and Voûte (1973), for example, are of the opinion that it is an illusion to think the diagnosis can be kept secret from the older child. But they have their doubts about the question to what extent the child should be actively informed about his or her illness. They write: "...the child does not ask many questions, but has all the more suspicions...We don't tell them everything, but we don't tell them fairy tales either. We have not yet dared to penetrate the heart of the matter. We feel one should not breach the defenses built up by patients around the disease." Issner (1973) emphasizes the central role of the doctor in the transmission of information to the child. If the doctor chooses a protective approach, the other hospital staff must adhere to this approach in order to avoid discord so as not to confuse the child. The behavior of doctors and hospital staff is an important example for the parents. Johnson et al. (1979) also point out that the way the doctor informs the child about the diagnosis sets the stage for the communication style chosen by the parents. Encouraging open communication between parents and child and demonstrating the beneficial effects of open communication is commendable, according to Spinetta (1978), but should not be forced. Especially in the initial stage, a temporary denial can be beneficial in order to enable a person to cope with the shock. Those who favor open communication with the child, seldom discuss the issue whether a child should be informed of his or her impending death. Nitschke et al. (1982) report their experiences with a policy of openly informing children who have reached the dying stage. They indicate that children can cope with knowledge of their impending death. Spinetta (1980), Spinetta and Deasy-Spinetta (1981), and Adams-Greenly (1984) provide a number of specific guidelines for hospital staff about how to talk about death with the child who has cancer.

Data on the parents' opinions about informing their child, or data on opinions of children with cancer themselves, are very sparse in the literature. In discussions with parents of children with cancer, Futterman and Hoffman (1973) often heard the opinion that knowledge of the fatal outcome of the disease would be destructive for the child. In their study, Koocher and O'Malley (1981) asked former pediatric cancer patients and their parents about their opinion on informing children about the diagnosis. Among the long-term survivors, 70% believed children should be told the diagnosis. Ninety percent of the parents shared this opinion and most of them thought this should be done immediately after diagnosis. A small number of parents (10%) felt that the diagnosis should not be told unless the child asks about it. Many parents themselves had not informed their child of the diagnosis because this had been discouraged at the time. Afterwards most of them deplored their lack of openness because, in their opinion, this had been a source of stress and difficulties, both during and after the child's treatment.

4.4. Empirical research into the communication processes of children with cancer

Few studies have been conducted on the communication processes of children with cancer. These are mainly directed at the provision of information about the disease to the child. Moreover, these studies show many methodological shortcomings.

Binger et al. (1969) interviewed the parents of 23 children who had died of leukemia, and report that only two children (adolescents) had been informed about the diagnosis by their parents.
In the repeatedly mentioned American study by Koocher and O'Malley (1981), 114 former pediatric cancer patients and their parents were asked questions about the provision of information. The authors only report the patients' data because the parents' answers deviate strongly from the patients'. According to the authors, the retrospective nature of the study and a selective memory of those interviewed are responsible for this finding. To the question when and by whom the patients had been informed about the diagnosis,

42% of the patients answered that they had been informed early (within one year after diagnosis or before six years of age if the patient was very young) by their parents or their doctor; 38% were informed later by their parents or doctor, and 20% had not received any information from doctors or parents but had stumbled on to it by accident from peers, nursing files, books, radio, or television. What is precisely meant by information about the diagnosis is not mentioned by the authors, but presumably it concerns the term cancer. In a Swedish longitudinal study, Márky (1982) interviewed the parents of 22 children with cancer (aged 2-18 years). Of these parents, 45% indicated they had informed their child about the diagnosis and 18% of the parents had not told their child anything about the disease. This last group involved children between 2 and 6 years of age. The remaining children were informed by their doctor and in half of the cases the parents were present at the time. The information about the diagnosis contained either the term cancer or the term tumor. Besides the parents, Márky interviewed 11 children between the ages of 6 and 18. Just like the study by Koocher and O'Malley, a discrepancy appeared between the data from parents and data from children. The parents of children older than 8 years (73%) all said they had informed the child about the diagnosis. The results of the children's interview showed there was a good correspondence between what the child knew about the diagnosis (cancer or tumor) and what the child had been told according to the parents. However, the children named the parents only as the source of information in half of the cases. Márky also asked the children how often and with whom they discussed the disease. In the initial period it appeared that almost all the children had someone with whom they could discuss the disease. For more than half of the children, the parents were the most important communication partner. The frequency of the child talking about his or her disease decreased sharply after the initial period. After a few months, none of the children talked about their disease very often. The children did not find it difficult to talk about the disease either in this stage or in earlier stages. All of the children said that talking about the disease was a positive experience.

With the aid of a questionnaire, 63 American adolescents with cancer (11-20 years old), were asked about preferred sources of information about the disease, about information sources available to them, and about what kind of information they need (Levenson et al., 1982). The hospital where these adolescents stayed pursued a policy to inform all cancer patients about their diagnosis. The study showed the doctor to be the most important source of information for the adolescents, and two-thirds of the adolescents preferred the doctor as the person to receive information from about their disease. Younger adolescents (under 16 years) more often preferred their parents as the source of information. Adolescents recently diagnosed, and adolescents with a relapse or recurrence, clearly showed less need of additional information. The authors assume that the use of avoidance as a coping response explains the diminished desire for information in patients going through a period of great vulnerability. Studying the same group and also applying a questionnaire, Pfefferbaum and Levenson (1982) investigated which questions the adolescents especially wished to be answered by their doctor. To them it was very important to receive answers to questions about the seriousness and duration of the disease, the chances of metastases, and what to expect if this should happen, to questions about the long-term consequences, and to questions about causes and prevention of cancer.

With the exception of the latter study, none of the studies paid attention to the reliability of the instruments. Besides methodological shortcomings, empirical research also shows deficiencies with regard to content. The emphasis lies on the provision of information about the diagnosis. Communication about the potentially fatal outcome of the disease and about the emotional experience have barely received any attention. These topics have been examined in studies on children with cystic fibrosis. Although these studies show many methodological shortcomings, they do show that communication about the prognosis and about emotions is problematic and is avoided in many families (Burton, 1975; Tropauer et al., 1970; Turk, 1964).

4.5. Empirical research into the relationship between communication about the disease and emotional reactions of children with cancer and their parents

A possible relationship between communication about the disease and emotional reactions in children with cancer and their parents has rarely been the subject of empirical research. The studies conducted in this area, however few, will be discussed in detail below.

Kellerman et al. (1977) carried out systematic behavioral observations among 7 children who stayed in hospital for a long period (an average of 88 days). The children (an average of 6 years old) were in an advanced stage of cancer and were being nursed in a laminar flow in the isolation ward during a long period. All children were informed about the diagnosis. The authors do not mention whether the poor prognosis had been discussed with the children. The behavioral observations were carried out by the nurses and involved the frequency with which the children spoke about their illness and the children's mood. The relationship between communication and mood turned out to be quite strong. Children talking most about their illness were least depressed. But the authors themselves notice that children who do not say much and thus do not talk much about their illness will be labelled as gloomy or depressed more quickly. Furthermore, the sample is very small.

Spinetta and Maloney (1978) tested the hypothesis that children who can speak freely about the diagnosis and prognosis within their family, cope with the disease more adequately. Sixteen children with leukemia and their mothers participated in the study. The children's age varied between 6 and 10 years and they all underwent outpatient treatment. A questionnaire intended to determine the openness of communication within the family was completed by the mothers. It contained the following questions: how much does the child know about the disease, what questions does the child ask, what answers do the parents give, what questions do the siblings ask, and what are the parents' answers to these questions. An adequate adjustment to the disease was determined as a low degree of defensiveness (defense scale), positive self-esteem (Family Relation Test), freedom to express negative feelings towards family members (Family Relation Test), and expression of closeness to the parents (distance measure of hospital play). An open family communication appeared to be related to a lower degree of defensiveness and a higher degree of positive self-esteem in the child, and to the experience of being closer to the father. The authors conclude that their results can be interpreted as a confirmation of their hypothesis that children cope more adequately with their disease if they have the opportunity to openly discuss the diagnosis and prognosis within their family. This conclusion should only be regarded as a tentative one. The sample is small and the operationalization of the concept of open communication about the diagnosis and prognosis has its limits. For example, it is unclear whether the child's knowledge of the disease originates from open communication with the parents. Moreover, the reliability and validity of the communication scale have not been ascertained. As the authors state, it is not certain that only the mother's judgment of openness is a valid judgment of the family's communication.

Koocher and O'Malley (1981) examined the relationship between the provision of information to the child with cancer and the emotional adjustment in the long-term among 114 patients who had survived their illness by many years. The operationalization of the concept of the provision of information has already been explained in the previous section. In section 3.6, it has been described how the emotional adjustment has been operationalized. The part of the study referring to communication has been described more completely in an article by Slavin et al. (1982). This study confirms the hypothesis that patients informed early about their diagnosis show a more favorable emotional adjustment than patients from whom the diagnosis had been kept a secret. Patients diagnosed at an early age (under 6 years of age) and informed about the diagnosis at that time, said they experienced it as if they had known it all along. Patients who were not informed about the diagnosis until later on, or had found out themselves later on that they had cancer, seemed to have greater difficulty integrating this information. Many of these patients felt cheated and shocked and were still angry with their doctor or parents. They showed more fear of the possible consequences of cancer and had more trouble believing in the reassurances offered to them. The merit of this study is that it is based on a large sample and an adequate reliability of the instrument used to measure emotional adjustment. It is interesting to see that a relationship between communication and emotional adjustment exists in a highly heterogenous group. Cancer was diagnosed in this group during childhood years (between 0 and 18 years). In this study the patients' age varies between 5 and 36 years (an average of 18 years) and the time elapsed between the diagnosis and the study varies between 5 and 32 years (an average of 12 years). The study has one disadvantage: the questions on providing information are related to events which, for many subjects, took place in the distant past. Relying this heavily on memory may cause distortions. The discrepancies between the data of the patients and the data of the parents (see section 4.4) must probably be partly attributed to it.

Research into the relationship between communication about the disease and the parents' emotional reactions is almost entirely lacking. One study has been conducted among 23 sets of parents whose child had died of cancer (Spinetta et al., 1981). Parents were interviewed who had lost a child 3 years ago at most. The study was aimed at the emotional adjustment of the parents and at factors influencing it. One of these factors was the communication of the parents with their child during the course of the illness. Open communication was determined as: the child's awareness of the illness, continuation of communication about the disease during the course of the illness, the child's initiatives in the communication, the child's questions on the prognosis, honest answers to these questions by the parents, and the parents feeling that they had told the child enough. Communication with the other children in the family was determined in the same manner and also examined as a factor. Besides a consistent philosophy of life and continual support from the partner or other important persons, an open communication with the child during the course of the illness also turned out to be an important positive factor in the parents' emotional adjustment after the child's death. The communication about the disease with the other children in the family did not show any relationship with the parents' emotional adjustment. Specific disease-related variables of the child or the passing of time after the child's death also did not have any influence. Although the researchers precisely describe their instrument and the interview is scored by independent raters, there are no details given concerning the reliability, and the operationalization of the concept of open communication can again be criticized. The parents' feeling that they have said enough to their child does not, for example, have to mean that the parents have openly discussed the poor prognosis with their child.

Although a small number of studies do not actually focus directly on the relationship between communication and emotional reactions, these studies provide data of interest for this topic. Thus Vernick and Karon (1965) and Karon and Vernick (1968) report their impressions of the effects of a clinical policy, directed at actively providing information about the diagnosis to more than 50 children with leukemia between the ages of 9 and 20 years. According to the authors, none of the children responded negatively when informed about the diagnosis. As soon as the children encountered an open attitude, they began to ask many questions about the precise nature of the disease, the possible treatment methods, and the prognosis. The children demonstrated an adequate adjustment to their illness and in the long-term no negative consequences of this clinical policy were observed either. In a few other studies it has been found that children who are openly informed about the prognosis are still able to remain hopeful and confident about their future, even if they are told that the prognosis is poor. The same applies to their parents. Mulhern et al. (1981) studied 25 children with leukemia (3 to 16 years of age) and their parents. They found that the children were more optimistic about their life expectancy than their parents and were considerably more optimistic than their doctor. In turn, the parents estimated their child's survival chances higher than the doctor. In the initial stage of the disease, the children and parents had been informed by the doctor about the statistical probability of achieving an initial remission (95%) and achieving long-term survival without recurrence of disease symptoms (40-50%). This information was repeated often in the initial period. All the children participating in the study were in remission for a period of 1 to 19 months. Probably the children and their parents, to some extent, gained their optimism from this fact. Susman et al. (1982) studied 16 children and adolescents with cancer (8 to 21 years of age) and their mothers. All the patients had a poor prognosis. Their illness had already reached an advanced stage. The patients and their parents were fully informed at the hospital about the disease and the low statistical probability of treatment effectiveness. Both the patients and the mothers seemed to be aware of the poor prognosis, yet they were not pessimistic about the future. Many expressed optimism regarding future plans. Finally, we would like to mention Nitschke's et al. (1982) report. The authors provide an account of a clinical policy in which children, for whom hope had been given up, and their parents participated in a 'final stage conference'. At this conference the doctor openly provided information on the child's precarious condition and impending death. An offer was made for a final experimental treatment or a palliative treatment at home. On the basis of impressions from the medical staff and/or family members, the authors conclude that a child can deal with the message of impending death. The open informational policy seems to promote communication in the family and only two of the 42 children (6 to 20 years of age) responded to the openness with a severe depression and behavior disorders.

4.6. Recapitulation

In the above, we gave a review of various opinions on the desirability of open communication with the child who has cancer. Although most publications appeared at a time when the survival chances for children with cancer were less favorable, our impression is that no consensus has been reached yet about the desirability of open communication with the child, and opinions on this subject still differ. At present, it is common practice in the Netherlands to inform parents about the diagnosis and prognosis of their child, but the development of more effective treatment methods and the resulting more favorable prospects have not led to openly informing the child as a matter of course. One of the reasons why a clinical policy in the area of communication with the child who has cancer has not yet been developed in the Netherlands is probably due to lack of empirical data on which a policy can be based. Research results concerning the relationship between communication about the disease and emotional reactions of the child and their parents point to a favorable influence of open communication on emotional experience, but the studies show quite a few methodological shortcomings. Furthermore, research has been focused almost exclusively on informing the child, while other aspects of communication have been neglected. The continuation of communication during the course of the illness, and the verbal and non-verbal exchange of information about emotions, although included by most authors in the concept of open communication, have rarely been topics for study. Our impression is that the clinical practice of doctors is to mainly leave it up to the parents to inform their child about the disease. Doctors usually do not give advice to the parents on the subject of communication with the child. Instead, they follow the parents' communication style with the child. The other hospital staff are also committed to the communication style used by the parents and the doctor. Herein lies an important reason for directing our study at the parents' communication style when examining the relationship between communication about the disease and emotional reactions of the children and the parents. What we mean by the concept of open communication is indicated in section 5.1.

When studying the relationship between communication about the disease and emotional experience of the child and parents, we realize that the situation of the child with cancer and of the parents is characterized by contradictions which probably have repercussions for communication. There are contradictions inherent in the nature of the treatment ('get sick' to get well), in the uncertain outcome of the disease (the child may live or may die), and in child-rearing (preparing for a future which may never come). It is plausible that these contradictions will be reflected in the communication about the disease. They can arise in both the verbal and non-verbal communication channels separately and between the communication channels. When a message is contradictory, the receiver has to make a choice between the sender's alternative intentions. The choice determines the appraisal and the emotional value of the message associated with this appraisal. When the receiver is aware of the contradiction in the message, the receiver may become confused because he or she does not know which meaning should be attributed to the message. In the literature, some contradictions in communication are called paradoxical messages. Popular examples of such paradoxical messages in family communication are: "Be spontaneous" and "You are too obedient". These types of paradoxical messages are different from ordinary contradictions because the possibility of a choice between the sender's different intentions is undermined. When someone is exposed to paradoxical messages for a long time, it is called a 'double bind' (Bateson et al., 1956; Watzlawick et al., 1967). A double bind entails a greater risk of disapproval or imposed feelings of guilt if it is pointed out - no matter how carefully - that there may be a distinction between what is perceived and what "ought" to be perceived (Watzlawick et al., 1967). In a description of communication patterns between cancer patients, family members, and doctors, Longhofer (1980) found remarkable paradoxes and double binds. In the literature on communication in families with a child who has cancer, Karon & Vernick (1968) describe the phenomenon 'conspiracy of silence'. It means that each family member is aware of the potentially fatal outcome of the disease and knows or intuits that this should not be discussed. In this situation double binds could arise between the family members. After all, it is not to be expected that the child, in such a situation, would openly ask the question: "Am I supposed to know that I might die of my disease or not?" Research into the relationship between double bind situations and emotional experiences has led to very divergent results (Bateson, et al., 1956; Beakel & Mehrabian, 1969; Dush & Brodskey, 1981; Kuiken & Hill, 1985; Mehrabian & Wiener, 1967; Sluzki & Veron, 1971; Smith, 1976). Lange and Van der Hart (1979) blame this on the different opinions of authors as to what the concept 'double bind' actually means. They point out that in spite of the problem of an inadequate definition of the concept, the effect of double bind phenonema in human interaction should not be underestimated. Effects of the double bind phenomenon are proved more convincingly in casuistic descriptions than in empirical reasearch. This seems to be caused by the difficulty of operationalizing this concept. The difficulty is chiefly generated by the implicit character of paradoxical messages. After all, the implicit part of the message is, by definition, not explicit, either for the receiver of the message or for the researcher (Kuiken & Hill, 1985).

5. Research design and instruments

5.1. Theoretical framework and the question of the study

From the above, it should be clear that open communication may favorably influence the emotional experiences of children with cancer and their parents. There is, however, no unequivocal empirical evidence on which a clinical policy can be based. The studies mentioned show too many shortcomings concerning the operationalization of the concept of communication, the sample size, the research method, and the reliability of the measures. Our research is focused on the question: Is there a relationship between the communication style of the parents, on the one hand, and the emotional reactions of the child with cancer and the parents, on the other hand? Is an open communication style related to less negative emotions and more positive emotions?

The conceptualization of communication as the process of verbal and non-verbal information transfer between persons (see section 4.1), is the starting point for the definition of the concept of open communication style as the transfer of factual information about the disease, the verbal and non-verbal transfer of information about the emotional experience, and the frequency of information transfer. We use Frijda's (1986) emotion theory as our starting point and regard the emotional reactions of the child and parents as the result of a process of appraisal of the situation. We assume that cognitive evaluations are mainly related to: responsibility for the situation, uncontrollability of the situation, uncertainty about the situation, and restriction of life-style (see chapter 2 and 3). We use the following research model.

Our research focuses on the communication style, the emotional reactions, the situational, and the intrapersonal factors. The situational meaning structure is an intervening variable which we do not directly include in our study.

72   Children with Cancer

Figure 5.1

The Research Model

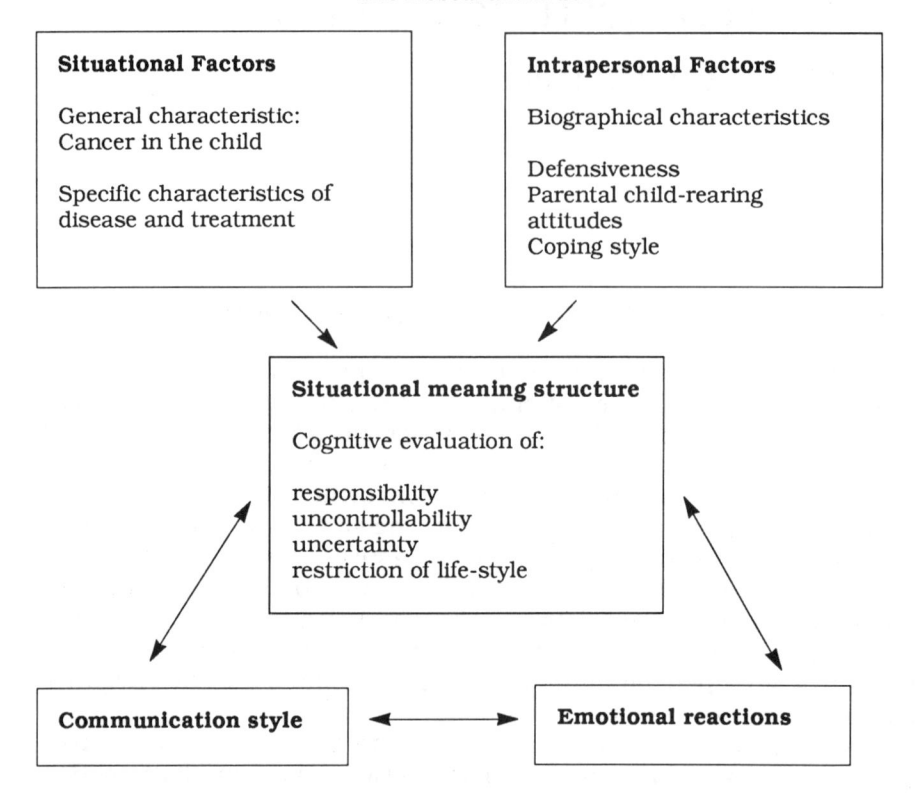

```
┌─────────────────────────────┐    ┌─────────────────────────────┐
│ Situational Factors         │    │ Intrapersonal Factors       │
│                             │    │                             │
│ General characteristic:     │    │ Biographical characteristics│
│ Cancer in the child         │    │                             │
│                             │    │ Defensiveness               │
│ Specific characteristics of │    │ Parental child-rearing      │
│ disease and treatment       │    │ attitudes                   │
│                             │    │ Coping style                │
└─────────────────────────────┘    └─────────────────────────────┘
              ↘                          ↙
              ┌──────────────────────────────────┐
              │ Situational meaning structure    │
              │                                  │
              │ Cognitive evaluation of:         │
              │                                  │
              │ responsibility                   │
              │ uncontrollability                │
              │ uncertainty                      │
              │ restriction of life-style        │
              └──────────────────────────────────┘
              ↙  ↑                        ↑  ↘
┌─────────────────────┐            ┌─────────────────────┐
│ Communication style │ ◄────────► │ Emotional reactions │
└─────────────────────┘            └─────────────────────┘
```

5.2. The research method

The hypotheses

The study is in three parts. In the first part we test our hypothesis; in the second part we give a detailed description of the communication process; in the third part we explore a number of relationships. The central question of our study leads to the following hypotheses which will be tested:
1. Children with cancer experience less negative emotions and more positive emotions if parents communicate more openly with the child about the disease.
2. Parents of children with cancer experience less negative emo-

tions and more positive emotions if they communicate more openly with their child about the disease.

It will be explored whether specific situational and intrapersonal factors influence both the communication style and the emotional reactions. The descriptive part of the study includes a detailed description of the communication style and the process of communicating about the disease in the family, at the hospital, and in the home environment. In the first and third part of the study we use the concept of communication style. By this we mean the factual information the parents have given their child about the diagnosis and the prognosis, the non-verbal information which the parents give their child about their own emotions, the information about emotions which the parents obtain from their child, and the frequency of communication about the disease between the parents and the child. The concept of open communication used in the hypothesis concerns the degree to which the parents use the mentioned aspects of the communication style towards their child. The study as a whole includes some more aspects of communication, namely communication about the disease within the family, at the hospital, and in the home environment. In discussing these data, we will use the more general term communication about the disease.

Subjects

A total of 82 children with cancer and their parents participated in the study. Families were selected on the basis of a stratified sample from the total patient population of children with cancer who are or were being treated in the Children's Oncology Center in Amsterdam, located in the Emma Kinder Ziekenhuis. In order to test our hypothesis in as wide an age group as possible, children between the ages of 4 years and 0 months to 16 years and 12 months were selected. We chose the age of 4 years as the lower limit because children of this age are considered to be capable of reflecting on their own behavior and the behavior of others and able to verbally express this reflection (see section 3.3). To optimize the representativeness of the sample, the following stratification criteria were used:
- age
- sex
- time since diagnosis
- prognosis

For the stratification of the criterion time since diagnosis, children were selected 4 months, 1 year, 2 years, and $3-3^{1/2}$ years after diagnosis. On the basis of the doctor's evaluation of the survival

Table 5.2.1
Distribution of the group according to age and sex

		girls	boys
Age	n	n	n
4	5	2	3
5	6	3	3
6	8	5	3
7	7	3	4
8	5	3	2
9	7	3	4
10	8	1	7
11	10	6	4
12	2	1	1
13	10	6	4
14	6	2	4
15	4	1	3
16	4	3	1
Total	82	39	43

chances of the child, the prognosis was indicated as good or poor. For a good prognosis survival chances were estimated to be greater than 50% and for a poor prognosis survival chances were estimated lower. By applying these stratification criteria, an optimal distribution was achieved in the group regarding age, sex, time since diagnosis, and prognosis. The distribution of the sample is presented in table 5.2.1 and table 5.2.2.

Data on the parents' education and socio-economic status of the family are reported in Appendix I. The age of the children and the parents, the size of the family, and the sick child's birth rank are also presented in Appendix I. The nature of the diagnosis and the status of the child's disease and treatment are reported in Appendix I as well. The geographical distribution of the group is large. The families come from eleven of the twelve provinces in the Netherlands. Of the 103 families who were asked to participate in the study, 21 families (20%) were not willing to participate. This number is rather high but is partially caused by the fact that the child as well as both parents had to be willing to cooperate in the study. Almost all parents who refused to cooperate gave the reason that the study would be too much of a burden for themselves and/or their child because they would again be confronted with painful experiences and emotions. These parents felt the need to

Table 5.2.2
Distribution of the group according to time since diagnosis and prognosis

Time since diagnosis	Prognosis		Total
	Good n	Poor n	n
4 months	14	6	20
1 year	11	11	22
2 years	9	11	20
3-3^1/$_2$ years	15	5	20
Total	49	33	82

distance themselves and "not to drag everything up again". The refusals bear no relation to the child's age, sex, time since diagnosis, or prognosis. Information was obtained from hospital staff who were familiar with these families about the communication style of the parents. There are no indications that refusals are related to a certain communication style in the family.

Procedure

Data collection took place between May 1983 and April 1984. The data were collected in the homes of the families. Prior to this, parents were informed by letter about the nature of the study. In order to avoid influencing the communication about the disease within the family beforehand, the purpose of the study was described as a study on the experiences of children and parents regarding the disease and the treatment in hospital. Parents were also informed about the procedure (interview, questionnaires, and play for younger children) and about the expected length of the interview (about 3 hours). A week after having sent the letter, the families were approached by telephone and asked if they would like to cooperate and make an appointment. During this conversation, it was checked whether the child's physical condition was such that he or she could participate in the study. Each family participating in the study was visited by three interviewers (the same persons each time) who interviewed and administered psychological tests to the child, the mother, and the father, separately and in different rooms. Prior to this, in a short joint introduction, the procedure was explained again. The interviews and tests were administered to the children by a female interviewer. The interviews and tests were administered to the parents by a male and a female interviewer. Fathers and mothers were equally distributed over both interviewers to avoid a systematic sex bias. The interview data were recorded on pre-coded questionnaires and on tape.

5.3. The instruments

Various methods of measurement were used for the operationalization of the different constructs in the research model. A major part of the selected instruments has been based on the method of self-report. This method is used for the children and the parents in a structured interview and questionnaires and it is also used in standardized play for the children. The disadvantages and limitations of self-report data are widely known in the social sciences: memory problems, the problem of social desirability or the desire of subjects to present themselves in a positive light, language ambiguities, and the problem of defense mechanisms. There are various ways to reduce and to some extent control the effect of these phenomena. The means used in our study towards this goal are explained below.

The choice of self-report as a method of measurement is based on a number of considerations. Firstly, subjective reports are the primary source of data about the quality of emotions (Lazarus & Folkman, 1984). What people say about their feelings and how they interpret what is happening to them are essential sources of information. The method of subjective reporting is also chosen for measuring the variable of communication about the disease. As there is no instrument available for measuring this variable, the communicative behavior of parents and children may be assessed by repeated behavioral observations. We decided not to choose this method because of the following considerations. First of all, it is to be expected that the frequency of occurrence of the relevant behavior will be low. An adequate sample of these types of behavior would require prolonged periods of observation which in actual practice would hardly be feasible. It should also be considered that the presence of an observer would probably interfere with the occurrence of this type of behavior. Moreover, important events taking place outside the observation periods or having taken place in the past cannot be discovered. On the basis of these considerations, it was decided to measure the variable of communication about the disease, as well as various other variables, with a structured interview.

The theoretical and empirical foundation of the concept of communication about the disease is still weak. The definition of the concept is still tentative and empirical relationships with other variables have hardly been studied yet. The interview method offers the opportunity to study a large number of potentially relevant aspects and relationships of the concept. Besides, this method offers the advantage of attuning the questions to the varying circumstances of our sample. In the next section we will describe the structure of the interview in more detail.

The problem of defense mechanisms connected to self-report methods was already pointed out above. This problem means that responses to questionnaires and interview questions cannot always be accepted at face value because a respondent can consciously or unconsciously deny negative experiences or emotions. This problem is very relevant to answering our question. Thus it is important to examine to what degree defensive appraisals and defensive modes of coping do occur in children and parents, and to what degree these will influence the test results. A self-report questionnaire, suited to this purpose, was used for the children. Such an instrument was not available for the parents. In addition to this, projective measures were developed by us for the children and the parents, based on the method of attributive projection (see De Zeeuw, 1976). This means that a person is asked to attribute thoughts, feelings, and behavior to others. The basic assumption of this method is that the person's own - perhaps defensive - thoughts, feelings, and behavior are projected onto the other person. Projective methods as indirect measures are distinguished by De Zeeuw (1976) from direct methods on which the self-report methods are based. This division will be used in the discussion of the instruments in the following sections.

First we would like to mention a number of general considerations made when selecting the instruments. First of all, this concerns the endeavour to measure the variables with already existing reliable and valid measures. Another criterion is the applicability of instruments for our specific population and especially for the children who form a heterogenous group with regard to age. To improve the comparability of test data for children in different age groups, instruments were chosen as much as possible on the basis of their applicability to a wide age range. On the one hand, the demands that the instrument makes on the young child's linguistic skills and abilities of abstract thought had to be taken into account and, on the other hand, the language used must not be too infantile for the older child. In the process of selection, instruments were preferred which had already been tested by other researchers in comparable populations of ill children. For those variables for which no adequate instruments were available, we designed our own measures. Scale analyses were conducted on these instruments. Furthermore, scale analyses were conducted if an instrument was used for a different age group than the one for which the instrument had originally been developed. Results of these scale analyses are reported in the description of the separate instruments. The statistical procedures used are set out in section 5.4. The test battery for parents and/or children has been composed of instruments to which the following research methods have been applied.

Direct measures:
- Structured interview
- Self-report questionnaires
- Standardized play
- Q-sort

Indirect (projective) measures:
- Standardized play
- Q-sort
- Response time

When selecting and designing the instruments and in choosing the order of presentation, an attempt has been made to introduce such a variation of research methods that the attention and motivation of children and parents should be stimulated as much as possible. One reason for this is to reduce the potentially threatening nature of the research situation, especially for the younger children. Separate test protocols were made for the children and parents in which all the instruments and instructions were included, except the questionnaires. The test protocols are available from the authors.

The instruments are discussed separately in the following sections. They are arranged according to the variables measured, using a subdivision of instruments for children and for parents and a subdivision of direct and indirect measures. Because not all instruments were used in all age groups, the number of children to whom the test was administered is reported each time. For the instruments used for the parents, the number of parents is equal each time. It concerns 159 parents: 81 mothers and 78 fathers. Before the description of the separate instruments, the general design of the interview for children and parents is explained in more detail.

General design of the interview

A structured or standardized interview was chosen for both parents and children. In this type of interview, the formulation of the questions and the order in which they are put to respondents are accurately recorded on paper and are the same for all respondents (Richardson et al., 1965). Standardization of the questions and the standardized way in which the interview is conducted serve the purpose of receiving the same information from all respondents. This makes an objective quantitative processing of research data possible. The questions partly consist of pre-coded questions and partly of open questions in which the initial answers are further clarified and amplified. In designing the interview, general rules were observed such as using clear, simple language and avoiding suggestive questions (Cannel & Kahn, 1953). A number of questions is not meant to be included in the data analysis. The function of these questions is to help respondents remember distant events, to direct their attention towards certain events, and sometimes also to reduce tension after emotionally loaded topics have been brought up. The interview is recorded on a cassette tape while it is being conducted. For children the interview is divided into two parts and for the parents into six parts. The topics included in the interview are discussed below, first those for the children and then for the parents.

The interview for the children

The interview for the children was developed for children from 8 to 16 years. The verbal and cognitive development of children under 8 years is still insufficient to allow us to interview them. Certain topics which are included in the interview with the older children are also included in the standardized play for the younger children. The interview contains the following topics.

Knowledge of the disease. The questions concern the nature and seriousness of the disease and are formulated in fairly general terms such as: "When you were in hospital, what was wrong with you?" and follow-up questions such as: "What else do you know about the disease?" Then the child is asked whether he or she still has the disease or is now definitely better, whether the disease was/is bad or serious, and why the child still has to be admitted to hospital or visit the clinic. The questions have been formulated in fairly general terms for ethical reasons. They do not guarantee that the knowledge which the children have about their disease is being completely tested. We have to proceed with caution because of the necessity to avoid giving the children information about their illness which they do not possess as yet.

Sources of information about the disease. A number of questions refer to the child's sources of information: from which persons the child has received information about his or her disease including the parents, doctor(s), nurses, fellow patients, siblings, and other persons inside or outside the hospital. It is asked what kind of information these persons have provided and in which period of the illness this happened. It is also asked whether the child noticed non-verbal expressions of worry and grief from the parents. The initiatives the child takes to gain information about the disease are also asked about, as are the questions he or she asked various persons, and the difficulties which he or she experienced doing this.

Communication about the disease with parents. The questions are related to communication about the disease with parents in the current period of illness, the child's main communication partner, who takes the initiative to communicate, and the need for and the appreciation of communication about the disease with the parents.

Communication about the disease with others. These questions refer to the content of the communication about the disease with fellow patients, siblings, classmates, and friends. There are also questions concerning the need for and the appreciation of this type of communication.

Positive and negative experiences in regard to the disease. Questions are asked about the most negative aspects of the disease and the positive and negative experiences during hospitalizations.

The interview for the parents

The interview for the parents includes the following topics.

Communication about the disease with the child. A large number of questions is concerned with the information about the disease the parent has given to the sick child, such as information given during the period of diagnosis, in the current period of illness, and during the periods in between. In the last part of the interview, detailed questions are asked about the information the parent has and has not given the child concerning the diagnosis and prognosis and in which period the information has been given. The questions also concern the frequency of communication with the child during the current period of illness, who takes the initiative in this regard, the questions the child asks about the disease, whether the parent expresses worry and grief in the presence of the child, and whether the parent asks about the child's worries and grief. Questions on communication with the child about fellow patients who died are also asked.

Communication about the disease with siblings. These questions concern the information about the disease which the parent has given to the siblings in the early and in the later stages of the disease, as well as questions the siblings ask about the disease.

Communication about the disease with the partner. The questions inquire about the frequency of communication about the disease with the partner, about appreciation of this, and about the initiator of communication.

Communication about the disease with parents of other children with cancer. The questions focus on the need for and appreciation of communication with other parents. Questions are also asked about participation in parent groups, appreciation of communication in these groups, and the need for participation in these groups.

Information which others have given about the disease. The questions concern the information about the disease which doctor(s) and others have given to the sick child and to the siblings.

Difficulties and emotions when communicating about the disease. These questions concern the difficulties the parent has when communicating about the disease with the sick child and with the siblings, the emotions experienced by the parent during the communication, and the control of emotions in the presence of the sick child.

Planning how to give information about the disease. The questions focus on the considerations which played a role for parents when informing the child about the disease, consultations which have taken place with the partner about this, advice obtained from the doctor(s), nurses, and psychosocial staff concerning informing the child, and the planning on how to give information about the disease to the child in future.

Controlling the information transfer about the disease. The questions concern the parent's worries regarding information about the disease which others could give to the child, actions which are taken by the parent to restrict information to the child including instruction to others not to give certain information about the disease to the child, restrictions which the parent places on him or herself when communicating about the disease with doctors, friends, and relatives in the presence of the child, measures to prevent the child obtaining information about the disease through printed matter or television, and instructing the sick child and the siblings not to pass on certain information about the disease to others.

Opinion on the child's awareness of seriousness. The questions focus on the parent's opinion regarding the child's awareness of the seriousness of the disease.

The child's behavioral problems. The parent is asked questions about the child's problems such as sleeping problems, eating problems, bed-wetting, problems at school, and problems in contacts with peers.

Optimism versus pessimism. The questions are directed at the parent's optimism versus pessimism on the chances of the child being cured in the initial period and in the current period of the disease, and thoughts about losing the child.

Information-seeking behavior. Questions are asked about activities undertaken by the parent to obtain information about the child's disease from doctors, by reading about the disease, by watching television, by consulting the instruction sheets included with medicines, and by visiting cancer information centers.

Inter-rater reliability of the interview data

Two independent judges have scored a random sample of 15% of the interviews with the children and 15% of the interviews with the parents. The inter-rater reliability is .94 for the interviews with the children and .92 for the interviews with the parents.

Emotional reactions of children and parents: Direct measures

The child's anxiety trait and anxiety-state

The STAIC A-Trait Scale (ST-AT). Anxiety trait or the tendency of the child to experience situations as threatening and to react to these with anxiety reactions is measured with the Dutch version of the Anxiety-Trait Scale (A-trait), a part of the State-Trait Anxiety Inventory for Children (STAIC) developed by Spielberger et al. (1973). This self-report questionnaire was translated and revised by Bakker and Van Wieringen (1985). The scale contains 20 items consisting of questions about the frequency of the child's cognitive, affective, and somatic manifestations of anxiety. The questionnaire is intended for children from 9 to 12 years of age. Reliability and validity of the A-trait scale are reported to be satisfactory (Bakker, 1981). The questionnaire was administered by us to 56 children between the ages of 8 and 16 years. Although the A-trait scale in the adult version (STAI) appears to be suitable for children from 12 years on (Van der Ploeg, 1981), we preferred to use the children's version for the older children too. The formulation of the items in the children's version also seems to be adequate for older children. Furthermore, the use of the same scale allows comparisons to be made between the different age groups. An item analysis was performed on the scale because data on the reliability of the questionnaire are only available for 11 and 12 year old Dutch boys (Bakker, 1981) and because the questionnaire was administered in our study to children in a wider age range. The reliability coefficients are .87 for the total group of children, .89 for the 8 to 12 year old children, and .88 for the 13 to 16 year old children. The internal consistency values are thus somewhat higher than the values reported by Spielberger et al. (1973) and by Bakker (1981). Thus we can conclude that the reliability of the questionnaire, for both the age group for which the scale was developed and for the older children, is very satisfactory.

STAIC A-State Scale (ST-AS). The Dutch version of the Anxiety-State Scale (A-state) from the State-Trait Anxiety Inventory for Children (STAIC) by Spielberger et al. (1973) is used to measure the child's anxiety-state. This scale was also translated and revised by Bakker and Van Wieringen (1985). The questionnaire contains 20 items concerning the actual anxiety reactions at the time the questionnaire is being completed. In this scale the questions concern the intensity of the child's cognitive, affective, and somatic manifestations of anxiety, and indicates the degree to which the child interprets the present situation as threatening. The scale can therefore be used to investigate to what extent the child experiences the interview situation and talking about the disease as threatening and anxiety-arousing. The reliability and validity of the A-state scale has been proven to be satisfactory (Bakker, 1981). The scale is intended for children from 9 to 12 years of age but in our study it is administered to 56 children from 8 to 16 years for the same reason as the anxiety trait scale. The item analysis resulted in the following reliability coefficients: .83 for the total group of children, .84 for the 8 to 12 year old children, and .83 for the 13 to 16 year old children. These values correspond closely to the internal consistency values from the study by Spielberger et al. (1973) and Bakker (1981), so that it can be concluded that this scale is also reliable when used for older children.

The child's depression

Depression questionnaire for children (DQC). The Depression questionnaire for children (version 4) has been developed by De Wit (1985) and is used for measuring depression manifestations in children. The questionnaire consists of 92 items and 20 dummies. Dummies are neutral questions not related to depression, and are therefore not scored. They are intended to counteract induction of a depressive response set. The scale contains 9 subscales which measure affective, motivational, secondary, and previous depression manifestations. The subscales are described as: depressive mood (affective manifestations); a decrease, slowing down, or regression of functions and behavior (motivational manifestations); depressive manifestations in the past; secondary somatic symptoms; negative self-evaluations; negative evaluations of the social environment; negative evaluations of the future; negative evaluations-attributions; negative evaluations-pictures. The questionnaire has been developed for children from 9 to 12 years of age. The total scale has a very high reliability (.94) and the separate subtests also have a satisfactory degree of reliability. There is enough empirical support for the construct validity of the scale. In our study, the questionnaire has been administered, for the same reason as the anxiety scales, to 56 children between the ages of 8 and 16 years. The item analysis of the total scale resulted in the following reliability coefficients: .95 for the total group of children, .95 for the 8 to 12 year old children, and .93 for the 13 to 16 year old children. Besides the total scale, we used the following 3 subscales of the DQC in our study:

Subscale NE-se: Negative self-esteem; 15 items
Subscale NE-ese: Negative evaluation of social environment; 7 items
Subscale NE-f: Negative expectations for the future; 8 items

The reliability coefficients of these subscales are: .76 (.76); .58 (.67); .71 (.62), respectively. The values in brackets are the reliability coefficients found by De Wit (1985). The reliability coefficients of the total scale and the subscales are high enough to use the scales in our study.

The child's emotional experience of the family relations

Family Relations Test (FRT). The child's affective relations with various family members is measured by the Family Relations Test (FRT). The English version was designed by Bene and Anthony in 1957 and was adapted in 1978. A Dutch version of the FRT, including preliminary population norms, was published by Baarda et al. (1983). The test provides quantitative and qualitative data on the nature and intensity of positive and negative feelings of the child, in which a distinction is made between the child's feelings towards other family members and the feelings of the other family members towards the child. Here family relations are involved as perceived and experienced by the child. The test also provides information on the young child's dependence or overprotection by the mother, and overindulgence of the parents towards the older child. The research method used in this test is based on the technique of standardized play. There are two versions of this test: one for younger children from 4 to 6 or 8 years consisting of 40 items, and one for older children from about 6 to 16 years containing 86 items. From a number of figures drawn on cards, the child chooses those figures which represent the family members. A box is attached to these drawn figures into which the child deposits the items printed on card. Psychometric data of the Dutch version of the FRT are available to a limited extent only for now. The test is not designed for determining the internal consistency because the scores are not mutually independent. This necessitates research on the stability of the test. However, repeating the measurements for determining the reliability lies outside the scope of our study. The test-retest reliability of the English version has been examined several times and proven satisfactory. The reliability coefficients range from .70 to .90 (Bean, 1976). There is still a lack of data with regard to the validity of the test. Few validation studies have been conducted and they are mostly directed at discrimination towards emotionally disturbed children. These studies have provided contradictory results. Bean (1976) doubts whether the FRT can be used as a measure of emotional adjustment which could be validated by a comparison with behavioral assessments. According to Bean, the FRT should be conceived as a measure of subjective perception of affective family relations. Consequently that is the way the test is used in our study. The version for younger children was administered to 26 children from 4 to 7 years of age; the version for older children to 56 children from 8 to 16 years of age.

Psychological and psychosomatic stress reactions and anxiety-state of the parents

Well-being scale: psychological stress reactions (W-P) and psychosomatic stress reactions (W-PS). Psychological and psychosomatic stress reactions in the parents are measured with a short version of the N and NS scale from the Amsterdam Biographical Questionnaire (ABQ) developed by Wilde (1970). The N scale measures psychoneurotic symptoms and the NS scale measures neurotic-somatic symptoms. The reliability and validity of these ABQ scales are reported to be satisfactory (Wilde, 1970). Jessen (1974) selected items on the basis of the highest factor loadings resulting in an N scale of 8 items and an NS scale of 14 items. These scales were used in a study by Jessen (1974) and in a follow-up study by Ormel (1980a, 1980b). Ormel called the scales the Well-being scales. The internal consistency of the scales in this short version was found to be moderate (the reliability of the N scale ranged from .69 to .76; the NS scale from .64 to .77). The stability of the scales turned out to be surprisingly good, even over a period of 7 years. This fact and other research findings by Ormel (1980a, 1980b) indicate that the scales measure a relatively stable personality trait, namely feelings of well-being which are predominantly dispositions of a person. According to Ormel, the scales measure the person's tolerance for and reactions to problems and disturbing events. Based on the above findings, we consider the Well-being scale for parents suitable for use in our study. We call the subscales the Well-being scale for psychological stress reactions (W-P) and the Well-being scale for psychosomatic stress reactions (W-PS). Considering the burden which the parents of a seriously ill child have to bear, we do not think it is fair to label these as neurotic symptoms. We prefer the term stress reactions.

Self-Report Questionnaire (SRQ-AS). The parents' transitory emotion of anxiety, also called state anxiety, is measured by the Self-Report Questionnaire Anxiety-State (SRQ-AS) of Van der Ploeg et al. (1980). The questionnaire is a Dutch version of Spielberger et al.'s (1970) State-Trait Anxiety Inventory. The scale contains 20 items measuring the intensity of feelings of tension, restlessness, anxiety, and nervousness which a person experiences at a given moment. The scale is very suitable for determining the effect of stressful events. The scale's reliability is adequate with reliability coefficients ranging from .93 to .96 (Van der Ploeg, 1981). The validity data reported by Van der Ploeg et al. (1980) and Van der Ploeg (1981) indicate that the scale is a valid instrument for measuring temporary increases in anxiety level caused by a condition which is experienced by the individual as stressful and threatening. Thus the questionnaire seems suitable for examining to what extent parents experience the interview situation as threatening and anxiety-arousing when emotional topics are brought up, such as their child's disease and communication about the disease with their child.

Pessimism about the course of the illness (PI)

Three questions in the parents' interview focus on pessimism about the course of the child's illness. The parents are asked whether they were optimistic or pessimistic about the chances of a cure for their child in the current stage of the disease; whether they think about losing their child, and if so, whether they think about this everyday or not. The reliability coefficient resulting from the item analysis is .86, making the scale's reliability adequate.

Use of sleeping pills and sedatives (MC-S) and the frequency of visits to the family doctor (MC-D)

The parents' emotional problems can become evident from the use of sleeping pills and sedatives and visits to the family doctor, also called medical consumption (MC). The parents are asked the following questions: "Have you used sedatives or sleeping pills during the past week?" and "How often have you seen your doctor during the past three months for your own complaints?

Assessment of the child's emotional behavior by the parent

Behavioral assessment scale for the parent (BAP). In order to determine the parents' view on emotional behavior displayed by the child, a checklist analogous to the semantic differential technique developed by Osgood et al. (1957) was constructed by us. On thirty-five 7-point scales, the parent indicates how the sick child has been behaving lately. On this behavioral assessment scale for the parent (BAP), opposite behavioral dimensions are mentioned at each pole of the scale, for example, cheerful-gloomy. The behavioral dimensions in these bipolar scales were chosen on the basis of emotional behavior of children with cancer, reported in the literature. Relevant behavioral dimensions used by Kamphuis (1976) in a study on children with cardiac disease were also chosen. Moreover, behavioral dimensions which could bear a direct relationship with the communication style of the parents were also included, for example, openness versus introversion of the child. The item analysis of all the scales resulted in a reliability coefficient of .93. After factor analysis, four main dimensions were selected as subscales. These are:

Subscale BAP-CR: Calm versus rebellious behavior. The scale contains 11 behavioral dimensions: calm-excited; cooperative-noncooperative; cautious-incautious; modest-demanding; easygoing-difficult; obediant-rebellious; contented-discontented; wait-and-see/demanding attention; not aggressive-aggressive; patient-impatient; peaceful-quarrelsome. The reliability coefficient of this scale is .91.

Subscale BAP-ChD: Cheerful versus depressive behavior. The scale contains 8 behavioral dimensions: optimistic-pessimistic; strong-weak; stable-unstable; happy-unhappy; confident-insecure; cheerful-gloomy; not lonely-lonely; high spirited-sad. The reliability coefficient of this scale is .87.

Subscale BAP-OI: Open versus introvert behavior. The scale contains 5 behavioral dimensions: talkative-quiet; sociable-withdrawn; assertive-shy; open-close; extravert-introvert. The reliability coefficient of this scale is .82.

Subscale BAP-NA: Not anxious versus anxious behavior. The scale contains 3 behavioral dimensions: not anxious-anxious; relaxed-tense; not nervous-nervous. The reliability coefficient of this scale is .71.

The reliability of the subscales were proven to be satisfactory and therefore the scales can be used in our study.

Problem behavior assessment scale for the parent (PBAP). Besides the aforementioned emotional behavior of the child, questions about the parents' view on specific problem behavior of their child were included in the interview for the parents. The questions in this problem behavior assessment scale for the parent (PBAP) are about actual behavior which can be seen as expressions of the child's emotional problems. These involve sleeping problems, eating problems, bed-wetting, problems at school, and problems in contacts with peers. Because the construction of a homogenous scale was not the goal when designing this part of the interview, an item analysis of items in each problem area sufficed. This resulted in the selection of the following subscales:

Subscale PBAP-SL: Sleeping problems. The 5 items in this scale refer to falling asleep, sleeping on and to the child's nightmares. The scale's reliability coefficient is .70.

Subscale PBAP-B: Bed-wetting. The 2 items in this scale refer to the occurrence and frequency of bed-wetting by the child. The intercorrelation of the items is .87.

Subscale PBAP-E: Eating problems. The 3 items in this scale refer to the child's habit of eating excessively or not eating enough, and to conflicts arising on account of the child's eating habits. The scale's reliability coefficient is .78.

Subscale PBAP-SC: Problems at school. The 3 items in this scale refer to the motivation of the child for going to school and to the child's school absenteeism which is not caused by the disease. The scale's reliability coefficient is .54.

The reliability coefficients of the subscales are in the acceptable range and therefore these scales are appropriate for use in our study. The intercorrelation of the questions referring to contacts with classmates and friends is not strong enough and therefore this subscale is omitted from the quantitative analysis.

Emotional reactions of children and parents: Indirect measures

Projection of situation-specific emotional reactions by the child

Hospital Play (HP). For young children, the applicability of direct methods of measurement is limited. Interview and questionnaire methods are not suitable for them. A hospital play was used to replace these methods of measurement for the young children (4-7 years) and as a supplement for the somewhat older children (8-12 years). Spinetta (1972) used a similar play in studies among children with cancer. In a pilot study conducted by us, the hospital play appeared to be very suitable for children with cancer between the ages of 4 and 12 years (Wijmans-Bruggeman, 1981). The play consists of a replica of a hospital room. It is made of wood and has the following dimensions: length 50 cm., width 35 cm., height 30 cm. There are 3 walls with a window in each wall. The room is open at the front and the top. The floor is divided into 80 sections. The wooden dolls belonging to the play fit into openings in these sections. These dolls represent the following figures: a child, a mother, a father, a doctor, and a nurse. There is a bed, a small cupboard, and a large cupboard in the room. The method of the hospital play can be characterized as a projective test employing a structured interview method. The play begins with an explanation that the doll is in hospital and must remain in bed. The child is asked to give the doll a name. The doll keeps this name for the rest of the play. Questions are then asked about the doll. These questions concern the nature and seriousness of the disease, the experiences in hospital, and the thoughts and feelings which accompany these experiences. The other dolls are introduced into the play, one by one, and questions are asked about the events which take place, about communication taking place between the figures, and about the feelings they experience. The statements made by the child about each one of the dolls are conceived to be a projection of the child's own experiences, thoughts, and feelings. The hospital play was administered to 58 children between the ages of 4 and 12 years. The child's answers were recorded on tape and the tape was completely transcribed for scoring purposes. The starting point for the content analysis of the verbal material was Waechter's (1971) adjusted scoring system of McClelland et al. (1958), which was also used by Spinetta (1972). In the scoring system used by us, the statements of the children were analysed according to the following categories. Statements belonging to the category loneliness and isolation are, for example: "wanting to go home" and "wanting the parents to remain at the hospital". We found a high inter-rater reliability in our pilot study. Because the score of a category is influenced by the total verbal production of the child during the play, the scores are adjusted accordingly. The inter-rater reliability was determined using the adjusted scores. Two independent judges scored a random sample of 25% of the protocols. The reliability coefficients are mentioned below per category, in brackets. These categories are:

HP-LI: Loneliness and isolation (.96)
HP-FP: Fear of pain and procedures (.97)
HP-F : Frustration (.90)
HP-DA: Diffuse anxiety (.89)
HP-G: Grief (.98)
HP-P: Positive feelings (.95)

Considering the high inter-rater reliability coefficients, the categories are used as separate scales in the quantitative analysis of the study.

Instructional booklet for children (IBC). In addition to the direct measurements of anxiety and depression, we also applied indirect measurements of situation-specific emotional reactions of the 13 to 16 year old children in the study. A projective test based on the method of Q-sort was developed. In this test, descriptions of feelings that children with cancer could experience have been printed on 36 cards. The emotional reactions reported in the literature on children with cancer and our clinical experience with these children, provided the basis for describing these feelings. It involves anxiety and grief, feelings of pessimism, loneliness and isolation, feelings of helplessness, anger, shame, doubt, and positive feelings. We attempted to formulate the items in such a manner as to give expression to the situation-specific character of the feelings. Examples of the items are: fear that you will have to be admitted into hospital again; feeling bad about looking different because of the treatment; the feeling that treatment is never going to end; anger when you see what others get worked up about; the feeling that no one understands what you have to go through; enjoying the fact that you are being pampered. The test gets its projective form by the instruction. The children are asked to indicate the feelings which they think other boys and girls with the same disease have, and they are being requested to do this for the purpose of developing an instructional booklet for children in hospital. The children sort the cards according to what they consider to be the frequency of these feelings in others (almost all the time, often, sometimes, never). Sorting the items is done without requirements for the distribution across the response categories. The test has been administered to 24 children between the ages of 13 and 16 years. The item analysis resulted in a reliability coefficient of .92 for the total scale. Because the number of children tested (n=24) is not very high when compared to the number of items in the test, a cluster analysis was performed. Three subscales could be selected after the cluster analysis:

Subscale IBC-AF: Anxiety and frustration. The scale consists of 12 items and has a reliability coefficient of .91.
Subscale IBC-P : Pessimism. The scale consists of 2 items with an intercorrelation of .45.
Subscale IBC-LI: Loneliness and isolation. The scale consists of 3 items and has a reliability coefficient of .85.

The reliability coefficients of these three scales are high enough to use the scales in our study. The positive feelings did not form a reliable subscale. That is why positive feelings of the children in the age group 13 to 16 years could not be included in the study.

Indirect expressions of anxiety and tension by the child

Latency (LAT) and blocks (BLOCK). In addition to actual content, verbal responses contain other properties which may indicate the anxiety experienced by a person. For example, hesitations and silences during conversation are not only the result of cognitive information processing, but also of stress and anxiety which are assumed to interfere with these processes. Many experiments have proven that a positive relationship exists between silences during conversation and anxiety (see surveys by Murray, 1971 and Dechert & Raupach, 1980). Latency and blocks during the hospital play and the interview are defined by us as two indirect measures of the children's anxiety. Spinetta (1972) applied the same mea-

sures in an identical manner to children with leukemia and interpreted them as expressions of anxiety in response to emotionally disturbing questions (disease, hospital, etc.). Latency is the number of seconds between a standard question by the interviewer and a response from the child. The duration of the silence between question and answer is recorded with a stopwatch and scored as follows:
1 = latency of 6-9 seconds; 2 = latency of 10-14 seconds; 3 = latency of 15 seconds or more.
A block is the total absence of a verbal response to a standard question, or an answer which only consists of: "I don't know". Each answer given by the child, no matter how inadequate, and each answer given even after 15 seconds is not scored as a block. The answer: "I don't know that" is not scored as a block either. The total scores of latency and blocks during the hospital play and the interview were determined by using the tape recordings of both. In the hospital play, latency (LAT-HP) and blocks (BLOCK-HP) of 58 children between the ages of 4 and 12 years were recorded. In the interview, latency (LAT-ITW) and blocks (BLOCK-ITW) of 56 children between the ages of 8 and 16 years were recorded.

Projection of situation-specific emotional reactions by the parents

Instructional booklet for parents (IBP). In addition to the directly measured anxiety and psychological and psychosomatic stress reactions of the parents, the emotional reactions have also been operationalized in an instrument which indirectly measures the situation-specific emotional reactions of the parents. This is a projective test based on the method of the Q-sort and is similar to the instructional booklet for children. Descriptions of feelings are printed on 43 cards which parents of a child with cancer may experience. When describing these feelings, we were guided by the emotional reactions, reported in the literature, of parents with children who have cancer and our own insights based on clinical experience with these parents. It concerns feelings of anxiety and insecurity, loneliness and isolation, feelings of helplessness, grief and doubt, feelings of guilt, anger, and also positive feelings. An attempt has been made to formulate the items in such a way that they would express the situation-specific nature of these feelings. Examples of the items are: uncertainty about the outcome of the illness; grief because your child must undergo such unpleasant treatment; anger because it's your child who must suffer this fate; fear that you will lose the child; the feeling that no one understands what you have to go through; the feeling that you are able to realize that all things are relative. Here too the test gets its projective form by the instruction. The parents are requested to state which experiences, in their opinion, other parents of a child with cancer may have and they are told this request is made for the purpose of writing an instructional booklet for parents in the hospital. Parents sort the cards according to how often they think other parents experience these feelings (almost all the time, often, sometimes, never). Sorting the items is done without any requirements as to the distribution across the response categories. The item analysis resulted in a reliability coefficient of .93 for the total scale. After factor analysis, 5 separate subscales could be selected.

Subscale IBP-LI: Loneliness and isolation. The scale contains 10 items and has a reliability coefficient of .87.
Subscale IBP-AI: Anxiety and insecurity. The scale contains 7 items and has a reliability coefficient of .82.
Subscale IBP-P : Positive feelings. The scale contains 6 items and has a reliability coefficient of .80.
Subscale IBP-H: Helplessness. The scale contains 5 items and has a reliability coefficient of .77.
Subscale IBP-FK: Fear of not being able to keep it up. The scale contains 3 items and has a reliability coefficient of .71.
Subscale IBP-G: Feelings of guilt. The scale contains 2 items with an intercorrelation of .48.

The instrument has an adequate reliability which justifies its use in our study.

Communication about the disease

Information questionnaire for the child (IQC). A questionnaire developed for a previous study conducted on adolescents with cancer (Last et al., 1979) was administered to 56 children between the ages of 8 and 16 years in this study. The information questionnaire (IQC) contains 12 items with questions on the sources of information available to the child; on problems the child experiences when trying to obtain information about the disease from others and when talking about the disease with others; and on the child's need to be informed about the disease and the need to talk with other people about the disease. Examples of these items are: When I ask questions about my illness, I usually get an honest answer; I find it hard to talk about my illness; I want to know everything about my illness. The item analysis performed on the entire scale resulted in a reliability coefficient of .74, after 3 items were removed. The factor analysis resulted in a selection of 3 separate subscales, which can be described as follows:

Subscale IQC-SI: Sources of information. The scale contains 5 items and has a reliability coefficient of .64.
Subscale IQC-IO: Information obstacles. The scale contains 2 items with an intercorrelation of .50.
Subscale IQC-NI: Need for information. The scale contains 2 items with an intercorrelation of .46.

Thus the subscales are reliable enough to be used as separate scales in the study.

Communication style of the parents with the sick child

Communication style of the parent (CSP). In the interview for the parents, 52 questions refer to various verbal and non-verbal aspects of communication about the disease between the parent and the sick child. The questions provide detailed data on the information which the parent has given the child about the disease and on other types of communication about the disease between parent and child. The questions can be divided into 18 unconditional items, or rather, questions which apply to the situation of all families, and 34 conditional items. The latter consist of questions which either do not apply to the situation of all families or can only be asked if a previous question is answered in the affirmative, the so-called follow-up questions. The 18 unconditional items include questions on:
– the specific information about the disease which the parent, or the doctor in the presence of the parent, has given the child.
– the point in time at which information is given, that is, shortly after diagnosis (during the first hospital admission) or at a later stage of the disease.
– the frequency with which the parent takes the initiative, in the current stage, to talk with the child about the disease.
– the frequency of the child taking the initiative, in the current stage, to talk with the parent about the disease.
– the parent's urging the child to keep the information about the disease a secret.
– the parent's expressions of worry and grief to the child.
– the parent asking about the child's worries and grief.
– restriction of communication about the disease between the parent and others in the presence of the child.
– taking measures to prevent the child receiving information from other sources.

The conditional items are related to the above topics as well as to situations in which the parent has or has not spoken to the child about a deteriorating condition or the death of fellow patients. An item analysis was performed on the 18 unconditional items. After removing 4 items, the scale had a reliability coefficient of .77. After factor analysis, 3 subscales were selected:

Subscale CSP-ID: Information about the diagnosis. This scale contains 5 items with questions about the information the parent has given the child about the diagnosis in the initial stage or in a later stage: the seriousness, the duration, the medical term (tumor/growth/leukemia), the term cancer, and the possibility of a relapse or recurrence. This subscale has a reliability coefficient of .73.

Subscale CSP-IP: Information about the prognosis. This scale contains 2 items with questions about the information the parent has given the child about the prognosis in the initial stage or at a later stage: the possibility that the child will not get better and the possibility that the child will die of the disease. The intercorrelation between these items is .93.

Subscale CSP-CE: Communication about the child's emotional experience. This scale contains 2 items with questions on the parent asking the child about worries and grief. The intercorrelation between these items is .42.

The remaining items do not form subscales and are included as separate variables in the quantitative analysis. The items involve the following topics:

Variable CSP-EW: Expression of worries by the parent.
Variable CSP-EG: Expression of grief by the parent.
Variable CSP-CIC: Frequency of current communication about the disease at the child's initiative.
Variable CSP-CIP: Frequency of current communication about the disease at the parent's initiative.
Variable CSP-IC: Indirect communication by the parent. This concerns the (un)restricted communication about the disease with others in the presence of the child.

In this way, the communication scale proves to have an adequate reliability and can be applied in our study.

Communication style of one of the parents or both parents. The emotional reactions of the child are tested for their relationship with the communication style of one of the parents or both parents. To achieve this, the scores of the above communication scales and communication variables of each pair of parents were converted into new scores in the following manner. When scores were not equal, the highest scores of one of the parents were used. When scores were equal, the scores of one parent were used.

The parents' attitude towards informing the child (AIP). In order to investigate the parents' attitude towards informing the child with cancer about the disease, we constructed an instrument based on the Q-sort method. Statements printed on 14 cards contain 7 items which refer to a positive attitude and 7 items which refer to a negative attitude towards informing the child. By sorting the cards, parents indicate if they agree with statements about positive or negative consequences if parents would fully inform children about their disease. The parents are instructed to think of children with cancer who are about the same age as their own child. Examples of the items are: If you would tell a child everything about the disease: -then a child would worry too much; -then a child knows he or she can trust you; -then this would make the child too anxious; -then a child knows that he or she can ask you all kinds of questions. There are no requirements as to the distribution of the items across the two response categories (agree - disagree). The item analysis of the total scale resulted in a reliability coefficient of .91. The factor analysis resulted in two distinct subscales:

Subscale PAI: Positive attitude towards informing the child. The scale contains 7 items and has a reliability coefficient of .91.

Subscale NAI: Negative attitude towards informing the child. The scale contains 7 items and has a reliability coefficient of .84.

Based on these results, the instrument can be considered reliable and suitable for use in our study.

Information-seeking behavior of the parents

Information-seeking behavior scale (ISP). In the interview for the parents, 18 questions are asked about the parents' activities to obtain information about the child's disease from doctors, their reading about the disease in newspapers, magazines, and books, their consulting medical journals and books and the instruction sheet included with the child's medicine, their watching television programs about this topic, and their visiting cancer information centers. These 18 questions form a scale with a reliability coefficient of .71, which is high enough to use the scale in our study.

Intrapersonal factors of children and parents

The child's defensiveness

Defense scale for children (DESC). The child's defensiveness has been measured by the Defense Scale for Children (DESC), developed by Dekking and Salentijn and described in Klomp et al. (1979). In this scale, defense is defined as the denial of anxiety and other unpleasant emotions and experiences which everyone has or has had at some time and which concern general and social situations. Thus the scale measures one aspect of defensiveness, namely the tendency of the child to deny negative emotions and experiences. The questionnaire contains 20 items and 8 dummies. The latter are neutral questions intended to disguise the content of the scale and to avoid response tendencies. These questions are not scored. Examples of items which measure defensiveness are: When you were little, were you ever afraid of anything? Have you ever been very angry? Do other children sometimes say nasty things to you? When constructing the items, an attempt was made to separate the concept of defense from the concept of social desirability and to formulate the items in such a way that a negative answer would indicate a strong distortion of reality and/or the child's own emotional experience. The items all refer to experiences which are universal for children or, put in another way, to experiences which cannot really be denied. The scale has been developed for children from 9 to 12 years of age and has an adequate reliability (KR-20 .82). The defense scale has a negative correlation (-.40) with the Social Anxiety Scale for children developed by Dekking (1983), and a positive correlation (.41) with the subscale Social Desirability in this test. These findings correspond with the results of Sarason et al. (1960), who studied the relationship between a similar defense scale and a test anxiety scale, as well as a general anxiety scale. Klomp et al. (1979) found further evidence for the construct validity of the defense scale from interviews with a few children. They found that children scoring high on the defense scale and low on the social anxiety scale use considerably more defensive coping strategies including rationalization, projection, and conscious denial of anxieties (social defense) than children who score low on both questionnaires. In our study the defense scale was administered to 56 children between the ages of 8 and 16 years. Some of the items on the defense scale contained the term *other children*. Because this formulation probably sounds too childish for the older age group, the term *other children* was systematically replaced by the term *other boys and girls*. The item analysis resulted in the following reliability coefficients: .86 for the total group of children; .85 for the 8 to 12 year old children; and .89 for the 13 to 16 year old children. The internal consistency values correspond highly with the internal consistency values found by Klomp et al. (1979). In spite of minor alterations and administration to children in a wider age range, the defense scale had an adequate reliability.

The parents' coping style

The Utrecht Coping List (UCL). We used the Utrecht Coping List (2nd version) developed by Schreurs et al. (1986b) to measure the parents' coping style. In this self-report questionnaire, coping is conceived as a relatively stable response style and a fairly consistent behavioral and cognitive response pattern in various problem situations. The content of the 47 items of the scale are related to four main categories of coping behavior:
a. behavior aimed at influencing the situation or otherwise, such as confrontation, avoidance, wait-and-see attitude.
b. behavior aimed at influencing the perception and evaluation of the situation such as optimism, acceptance, resignation, pessimism.
c. behavior aimed at reducing tension, the so-called palliative responses such as seeking distractions, smoking, and drinking.
d. expression of emotions.

Examples of some items are: Working towards solving a problem in a goal-oriented manner; Completely isolating yourself from others; Sharing your problems with others; Realizing that others could be having a hard time too. The questionnaire's instructions state that one indicates, on a 4-point scale, how often one reacts to problems or other unpleasant events in the manner indicated in the item. The Utrecht Coping List contains the following 7 subscales:

Subscale A: Active problem-solving; 8 items.
Subscale P: Palliative actions; 8 items.
Subscale Av: Avoidance and wait-and-see attitude; 9 items.
Subscale S: Seeking social support; 6 items.
Subscale D: Depressive reaction pattern; 7 items.
Subscale E: Expression of emotions/anger; 3 items.
Subscale C: Comforting cognitions; 3 items.

Three items of the questionnaire are not included in the subscales. The reliability coefficients of the separate subscales range from .62 to .82. Taking the small number of items in some subscales into account, the internal consistency of the scales can be called quite satisfactory. The form of the questionnaire (2nd version) used by us has undergone a few minor alterations in its final form. The reliability data (internal consistency and stability) of this final version of the scales is reported to be satisfactory, and a reasonable amount of empirical support for the validity has already been found (Schreurs et al., 1986b). One reason for using this questionnaire in our study is a pragmatic one. It is the only available and reasonably well-studied Dutch instrument for measuring coping, at least at the time we started our study. Another reason for choosing this questionnaire is that the operationalization of coping as a response style, i.e. as a personality dimension, is suitable for studying the relationship between the communication style of the parent with the sick child and the way in which the parent generally copes with problems. Should we find a relatively strong relationship and should the study give us reason to try and influence the communication style of the parents, then more intensive therapeutic interventions would be required.

The parents' attitude towards child-rearing

The Amsterdam version of the Parental Attitude Research Instrument (A-PARI). The attitude of the parents towards child-rearing is measured with the Amsterdam version of the Parental Attitude Research Instrument (A-PARI). It is a short version of the questionnaire originally developed by Schaefer and Bell (1958). Heydendael et al. (1979) have translated the questionnaire into Dutch and revised it, on the basis of psychometric and validity data from previous research, to a questionnaire consisting of 15 items. This short version was used by them in the Nijmegen Growth Study. The scale consists of four factors or subscales measuring different aspects of parental child-rearing attitudes. The structure of the factors corresponds to the four quadrants of Schaefer's (1959) theoretical model. The subscales are:
Subscale: Overprotection; 4 items.
Subscale: Autocratic attitude; 5 items.
Subscale: Autonomy-promoting attitude; 2 items.
Subscale: Self-pity; 4 items.
The items consist of statements such as: someday a child will be grateful for the strict upbringing you have given; a child is not allowed to have secrets from father or mother.
In the Nijmegen version of the PARI, each statement is followed by a 5-point scale. The same items are used in our study but each statement is followed by a 4-point scale. For this reason it is called the Amsterdam version of the PARI: the A-PARI. A reliability study and test standardization on the four subscales of the A-PARI was conducted by De Leeuw (1986). The subscales have the following reliability coefficients:
– Overprotection .67
– Autocratic attitude .77
– Autonomy-promoting attitude .55
– Self-pity .57

The reliability of the subscales is adequate, taking the small number of items per scale into account. Therefore the A-PARI can be used as a research instrument.

Biographical data of children and parents

Biographical data consist of sex, age, and birth rank of the child and the sex, age, education, and socio-economic status of the parents. The data were partly available from the child's medical records. The remaining data were obtained from the parents. The parents were asked about the birth rank of the child, their own age, the highest level of edu~iocation they started or finished, and their job or profession. The socio-economic status of the family was determined on the grounds of the highest educational level and job/profession of one of the parents. The criteria used by the Central Bureau of Statistics were applied. Data on the family's size and the age of the siblings were also obtained from the parents.

Situational factors of the child

Disease and treatment characteristics of the child

The following data were obtained from the child's medical records: nature of the diagnosis; time since diagnosis in months; treatment duration in months; undergoing treatment versus treatment finished; in initial remission; relapse or recurrence; in subsequent remission; frequency of clinic visits; number of hospital admissions; number of days in hospital; physical visible impairments as a consequence of the disease and/or treatment. As regards the latter, the data partly originate from the medical records, partly from observation by the interviewer, and partly from questions to the children and/or parents. The same criteria were used as in Koocher and O'Malley's (1981) study. They evaluated the degree of obviousness of physical impairments (obvious scars, deformities, baldness); the degree of interference with activities of daily living and of requiring help; the degree of physical dysfunction and need of medical attention or prosthetics; the degree of school absenteeism caused by the disease and/or treatment. The child's prognosis was evaluated by the pediatrician, as previously mentioned. A good prognosis is a survival chance greater than 50%; a poor prognosis is a survival chance less than or equal to 50%.

Outline of instruments for children and parents

Children
Emotion Variables

Parents
Emotion Variables

Anxiety scales   *Age group*

ST-AT	STAICAnxiety trait	8-16	W-P	Well-being scale psychological stress reactions	
ST-AS	STAICAnxiety state	8-16			
HP-FP	Hospital play: Fear of pain and procedures	4-12	W-PS	Well-being scale psychosomatic stress reactions	
HP-DA	Hospital play: Diffuse anxiety	4-12		Self-Report	
IBC-AF	Instructional booklet: Anxiety & frustration	13-16	SRQ-AS	Questionnaire Anxiety State	
LAT-HP	Latency Hospital play	4-12	MC-S	Medical Consumption Sleeping pills and sedatives	
LAT-ITW	Latency Interview	8-16			
BLOCK-HP	Blocks Hospital Play	4-12 / 8-16	MC-D	Medical Consumption Frequency of doctor's visits	
BLOCK-ITW	Blocks Interview		PI	Pessimism about course of illness	

Depression scales

Instructional booklet (IBP)

DQC	Depression questionnaire	8-16			
NE-se	Negative self-esteem	8-16			
NE-ese	Negative evaluation of social environment	8-16	IBP-LI	Loneliness and isolation	
NE-f	Negative expectations for the future	8-16	IBP-AI	Anxiety and insecurity	
			IBP-P	Positive feelings	
HP-LI	Hospital play: loneliness and isolation	4-12	IBP-H	Helplessness	
HP-F	Hospital play: Frustration	4-12	IBP-FK	Fear of not keeping it up	
HP-G	Hospital play: Grief	4-12	IBP-G	Feelings of guilt	
IBC-LI	Instructional booklet: Loneliness and isolation	13-16	*Behavioral assessment scale (BAP)*		
IBC-P	Instructional booklet: Pessimism	13-16	BAP-CR	Calm versus rebellious behavior	
			BAP-ChD	Cheerful versus depressive behavior	

**Children
Emotion Variables**

**Parents
Emotion Variables**

Positive feelings
HP-P   Hospital play:
        Positive feelings

Age group
4-12

BAP-OI   Open versus
          introvert behavior

*Emotional experience of
family relations*
Family Relations Test (FRT)
Positive feelings
towards:

BAP-NA   Not anxious versus
          anxious behavior

4-7
and
8-16

*Problem behavior
assessment
scale (PBAP)*

PM   Mother
PF   Father
PS   Siblings

PBAP-SL   Sleeping problems
PBAP-B   Bed-wetting
PBAP-E   Eating problems

Negative feelings
towards:

4-7
and
8-16

PBAP-SC   Problems at school

NM   Mother
NF   Father
NS   Siblings

Communication Variables
Information Questionnaire (IQC)

Communication Variables
Communication style (CSP)

IQC-SI   Sources of   8-16
          information
IQC-IO   Information   8-16
          obstacles
IQC-NI   Need for   8-16
          information

CSP-ID   Information about
          diagnosis
CSP-IP   Information about
          prognosis
CSP-CE   Communication
          about child's emo-
          tional experience
CSP-EW   Expression of worry
CSP-EG   Expression of grief
CSP-CIC   Communication
          about disease at
          child's initiative
CSP-CIP   Communication
          about disease at
          parent's initiative
CSP-IC   Indirect communi-
          cation

Children		Parents
Communication Variables	*Age group*	**Communication Variables**
		Attitude towards giving information (AIP)
		PAI — Positive attitude
		NAI — Negative attitude
		Information-seeking behavior scale (ISP)
Personal Factors		**Personal Factors**
Defense scale (DESC)	8-16	Utrecht Coping List (UCL)
		A — Active problem-solving
		P — Palliative actions
		Av — Avoidance and wait-and-see attitude
		S — Seeking social support
		D — Depressive reaction pattern
		E — Expression of emotions/anger
		C — Comforting cognitions
		Parental Attitude Research Instrument (A-PARI)
		Overprotection
		Autocratic attitude
		Autonomy-promoting attitude
		Self-pity

5.4. The statistical procedures

The results of the scale analyses have already been presented in the discussion of the instruments. The following statistical procedures were applied to these analyses. The inter-rater reliability of the scoring by two independent judges, performed on the protocols of the interviews of the child and the parents and on the protocols of the hospital play, has been calculated using the Kendall rank correlation coefficient (Siegel, 1956). The reliability of the scales, reported in section 5.3, has been calculated with the reliability coefficient Cronbach's alpha. The statistical program STAP (1980) was used for this calculation.

After an initial item analysis, items with an item-test correlation of <.20 were removed from the scale. The reliability of the scale was established again in a subsequent item analysis. The scale was only included in the quantitative analysis when the total scale had a Cronbach's alpha of >.70. Then a factor analysis was performed on the scales. The factor analysis is based on the VARIMAX method (SPSS program, 1981). This method consists of an iterative rotation of principal factors with an eigen value of 1.00 and higher (the eigen value is a measure of the explained variance). For one instrument, the children's Q-sort task (IBC), a Pearson cluster analysis type Elshout (STAP, 1980) was performed instead of a factor analysis because the proportion of items to subjects required this. The results of the factor analysis and the cluster analysis were checked for clustering of items with extreme p-values, but this did not appear to be the case. Another item analysis was performed on the subscales resulting from the factor analysis and the cluster analysis. In the final selection of subscales for the purpose of the quantitative analysis, the following limits were observed: Cronbach's alpha >.50 or intercorrelations >.40 whenever a subscale consisted of only two items.

For each instrument on which an item analysis and a factor analysis or cluster analysis was performed, the intercorrelation (Pearson correlation) was calculated between the sum scores of the subscales. The intercorrelations were also determined between scales which measure the same construct (communication, anxiety, depression) in various ways (directly and indirectly). The intercorrelations are reported in Appendix II.

The intercorrelations between the scales and subscales did not turn out to be high. This means that the concept of communication and the concept of emotional reactions each have different dimensions and cannot be conceived as unidimensional concepts. For this reason, the hypothesis about the relationship between the communication variables and emotion variables was tested separately for each subscale. For this reason, our intention to apply more advanced methods of statistical analysis was not feasible. The hypotheses were tested by a correlational method. The relationship between the communication variables and emotion variables was determined by calculating Pearson correlations.

We only assigned significance to the relationships when the number of significant correlations between the variables was greater than the 5% which can be expected by chance. We chose a significance level of 5% and a two-tailed test because a test result, even if contrary to our expectations, is also important due to the conclusion which should be drawn from it on behalf of clinical policy.

Partial correlations were calculated if a communication variable and an emotion variable were significantly correlated, while one or more situational factors or intrapersonal factors also correlated with both variables and might explain the relationship (see Ferguson, 1966). Pearson correlations and univariate variance analysis (ANOVA) have been applied to explore the effect of situational and intrapersonal factors on the communication variables and emotion variables. Student's t-test for independent samples has been used to examine differences between groups and subgroups. Within the sample, children in different age groups were compared to each other with regard to mean scores on emotion variables. The same comparisons were made between the group of mothers and the group of fathers. Comparisons with norm groups have also been made in this way.

The SPSS program (1981) has been used for calculating the Pearson correlations, partial correlations, t-tests, and univariate variance analyses.

6. Test of the hypotheses

6.1. The relationship between the parents' communication style and the child's emotional reactions

The child's emotional reactions have been studied according to their relationship with the communication style of one or both parents (see section 5.3). Because the child's sex has almost no influence on the parents' communication style, nor on the child's emotional reactions (see section 8.2), the statistical tests have not been performed separately for the boys and girls, but for the entire group of children. The relationship between the communication variables and the emotion variables of the child is tested by means of Pearson correlations. The tests show the following results:

- Children informed at an early stage by their parents about the nature and possible implications of their disease are less anxious, less depressed, have a more positive evaluation of their social environment, and display less behavioral problems than children informed later or almost not at all by their parents.
- The way the parents informed the child is not related to the child's positive feelings, nor to the way the child experiences the family relations.
- Communication about the emotional experience of the disease by the parents is not related to the child's emotional reactions.
- Children take the initiative to talk about the disease with their parents more often as they experience more negative emotions and display more behavioral problems.
- There is no unequivocal relationship between the frequency the parents take the initiative to talk to their child about the disease and the emotional reactions experienced by the child. If parents take the initiative to talk about the disease with their child more often, the child reports less anxiety and less depression. However, at the same time, younger and older children exhibit more tension, anxiety, and frustration under these circumstances.

- There is no unequivocal rlationship between the parents' indirect communication and the child's emotional reactions. When parents are used to talking freely with others about the disease in the presence of the child, the child displays less behavioral problems but exhibits more negative feelings.

These findings only partially support our hypothesis that an open communication style by the parents is associated with less negative emotional reactions and more positive emotional reactions in the child. Only with regard to the matter of informing the child about the disease do the results correspond with our expectations. With regard to the other communication aspects the relationships are either nonexistent or contrary to our expectations or equivocal. Moreover, it should be remarked that most of the relationships are not very strong, i.e. the correlations are not high.

In a number of cases, the relationship between the communication variables and emotion variables becomes somewhat stronger or even visible if the effect of the child's defensiveness is taken into account. The children's defensiveness or the children's tendency to deny anxieties and other unpleasant emotions and experiences which every child has or has had at some time, shows a distinct negative relationship with the anxiety, depression, and other unpleasant emotions children report and project. The communication style of the parents also has a weak negative relationship with the child's defensiveness. These relationships are explained further in section 8.3. Here we note that these findings constituted the reason for removing the effect of defensiveness from the relationship between the communication variables and emotion variables by calculating partial correlations.

In section 8.2 we describe the influence of biographical and disease characteristics on the emotional reactions of the child and the communication style of the parents. Whenever these variables correlate with both the emotion variables and the communication variables, this effect has also been removed by the use of partial correlations. The disease characteristics do not appear to influence the relationship found between the communication variables and emotion variables of the child in any way (the partial correlations are almost equal to the correlations). Barring one exception, the same applies to the biographical characteristics. We will discuss this exception below.

The means and standard deviations of the communication variables and emotion variables are presented in Appendix V. We did explore if it was important for the child's emotional experience that each of the parents should use the same communication style. We did not find any evidence of this. The mean scores on the emotion variables of the group of children whose parents used a congruous communication style did not deviate from the mean scores of the group of children whose parents used incongruous communication styles.

The results of the statistical tests are presented below in three groups. First of all, the emotional reactions of the child are related to the communication variables *information about the disease*; subsequently to the variables *communication about the emotional experience*; and finally to the variables *communication about the disease*. When relevant, qualitative data from the interview are used to illustrate the quantitative data. Instruments measuring the children's emotional reactions were not applied to the entire group of children, with the exception of the instruments measuring behavioral problems. In discussing the results, we will therefore indicate each time to which age group the results apply.

Information and emotional reactions

Information and the child's anxiety. Children who, in the initial stage of the disease, have received more information about the diagnosis and prognosis are less anxious than children who have received less information and/or information at a later stage.

Anxiety in the child has been measured in various ways: as a trait or tendency to experience anxiety, as an anxiety-state during the interview, when the disease and the emotional experiences associated with it are discussed, and as a projection of specific anxieties related to the disease. In addition, the parents assessed the degree of their child's anxiety. Table 6.1.1 presents the correlations between the anxiety variables of the child and the information about the disease given to the child by one or both parents. This table also presents the partial correlations. These indicate the relationship between anxiety and information, after the effect of the child's defensiveness has been removed. The number of significant correlations is greater than the 5% which can be expected on the basis of chance alone. The correlations and partial correlations are not high, but are nearly all in the expected direction. On the whole, it can be concluded that children who have received more information about the diagnosis and prognosis from their parents during the initial stage of the disease, are less anxious than children who have received less information and/or information at a later stage of their disease. This means that children are less anxious if they have already been informed about the nature and possible implications of their disease by their parents

Table 6.1.1
Pearson correlations (r) and partial correlations (part.r) between the communication variables "information about the diagnosis" (CSP-ID) and "information about the prognosis" (CSP-IP) on the one hand, and the anxiety variables of the child, on the other hand.

			Information given by the parents			
			about the diagnosis		about the prognosis	
Anxiety variables of the child	n'	n"	r	part.r	r	part.r
Direct measures:						
Anxiety trait (ST-AT) 8 to 16 year olds	56	56	-.18	-.28*	-.18	-.35**
Anxiety-state (ST-AS) 8 to 16 year olds	56	56	-.03	-.04	-.14	-.18
Anxiety assessment by the mother (BAP-NA) 4 to 16 year olds	81	55	-.34**	-.35**	-.17	-.18
Anxiety assessment by the father (BAP-NA) 4 to 16 year olds	78	52	-.29*	-.29*	-.22	-.23
Indirect measures:						
Latency (HP) 4 to 12 year olds	58	32	-.05	-.07	-.16	-.19
Latency (ITW) 8 to 16 year olds	56	56	.18	.16	-.15	-.21
Blocks (HP) 4 to 12 year olds	58	32	-.25	-.24	-.13	-.06
Blocks (ITW) 8 to 16 year olds	56	56	-.16	-.15	-.17	-.15
Projective measures:						
Fear of pain and procedures (HP-FP) 4 to 12 year olds	58	32	.09	.10	.02	.03
Diffuse anxiety (HP-DA) 4 to 12 year olds	58	32	-.26*	-.31	-.21	-.31
Anxiety and frustration (IBC-AF) 13 to 16 year olds	24	24	-.10	-.14	-.24	-.32

part. r = correlation between the variables after removing the effect of defensiveness
n' = size of sample when calculating the correlations
n" = size of sample when calculating the partial correlations
* = $p<.05$
** = $p<.01$

shortly after diagnosis, during their first stay in hospital. This involves the information that the disease is serious, protracted, is a type of cancer which may recur, and the information that the child may not get better or may die.

The values of the correlations show that the relationship is not a strong one. Furthermore, the relationship with information about the diagnosis is more evident than with information about the prognosis, although a similar trend can be seen here as well. The relationship has been found in all age groups: with the anxiety the child reports about him or herself (8 to 16 year olds), with diffuse anxieties which the child projects (4 to 12 year olds), and with the assessment by both the mothers and fathers about the child's anxiety (in all age groups). Because the sample size differs for each variable as correlations and partial correlations are calculated, the value a correlation must have to reach significance varies. The children's defensiveness is only measured in the 8 to 16 year old age group, therefore the partial correlations in table 6.1.1 only refer to this age group. On the whole, the existence of a relationship between giving information and the child's anxiety is somewhat more evident when the effect of the child's defensiveness has been removed. This applies to both the direct measures and the projective measures of anxiety. Considering that the sample size is small, the correlation has to be high to reach significance. That is why even a higher partial correlation is sometimes still not significant.

Information and the child's depression. Children who have received more information about the prognosis from their parents in the initial stage of the disease are less depressed than children who have received less information and/or information at a later stage. Children who have received more information about the diagnosis from their parents in the initial stage of the disease have a less negative appraisal of the social environment than children who have received less information and/or information at a later stage. Like anxiety, the child's depression has been measured in various ways using both direct and indirect (projective) measures. Furthermore, the parents have assessed the degree of the child's depression. Table 6.1.2 presents the direct measures of the depression variables. The correlations indicate the relationship of these variables with the information about the disease given by one or both parents to the child. The partial correlations are also presented. They indicate the relationship between depression and information after the effect of the child's defensiveness has been removed. The number of significant correlations between the communication variables and depression variables is greater than the 5% which can be expected on the basis of chance alone.

Table 6.1.2
Pearson correlations (r) and partial correlations (part.r) between the communication variables "information about the diagnosis" (CSP-ID) and "information about the prognosis" (CSP-IP) on the one hand, and the depression variables of the child, on the other hand.

			Information given by the parents			
			about the diagnosis		about the prognosis	
Depression variables of the child	n'	n"	r	part.r	r	part.r
Direct measures: Depression (DQC) 8 to 16 year olds	56	5	-.12	-.18	-.16	-.29*
Negative self-esteem (NE-se) 8 to 16 year olds	56	56	-.19	-.24	-.15	-.24
Negative evaluation of social environment (NE-ese) 8 to 16 year olds	56	56	-.28*	-.28*	-.24	-.24
Negative expectations for the future (NE-f) 8 to 16 year olds	56	56	.02	-.01	-.14	-.22
Depression assessment by mother (BAP-ChD) 4 to 16 year olds	81	55	-.16	-.19	-.13	-.18
Depression assessment by father (BAP-ChD) 4 to 16 year olds	78	52	-.11	-.14	-.15	-.21

part.r = correlation between the variables after removing the effect of defensiveness
n'   = sample size when calculating the correlations
n"   = sample size when calculating the partial correlations
*   = p<.05

On the whole, there is a slight negative relationship. This means that children who have received more information about the diagnosis and prognosis from their parents in the intial stage of the disease are less depressed and have a less negative evaluation of the social environment than children who have received less information and/or information at a later stage. From the values of the correlations, we see that the relationship is not strong. The significant relationship between depression and information about the prognosis does not become evident until the effect of the child's defensiveness has been removed. However, the latter does not influence the relationship between information and a negative evaluation of the social environment.

The relationship between depression and information only occurs in the 8 to 16 year old children and only with respect to the direct measures of depression. With regard to the projective measures of depression which have also been applied to the younger children, most correlations are slightly negative but not significant. This means that the projection of feelings of loneliness and isolation, feelings of frustration, and feelings of grief by the 4 to 12 year old children, as well as the projection of feelings of loneliness and isolation and feelings of pessimism by the 13 to 16 year old children is not related to the way parents informed the child about the disease. As we can see in Table 6.1.2, the parent's assessment of their child's depression is also not significantly related to how the parents gave information about the disease.

Information and the child's behavioral problems. Children who have received more information about the diagnosis and prognosis from their parents in the initial stage display less behavioral problems than children who have received less information and/or information at a later stage.

The child's behavioral problems are operationalized as the two behavioral dimensions: calm versus rebellious behavior and open versus introvert behavior. At the same time, they consist of several types of specific behavior which can be seen as expressions of the child's emotional problems, namely sleeping problems, bed-wetting, eating problems, and problems at school. The parents have assessed these problems of their child. The number of significant correlations between the communication variables *information about the disease* and the variables *behavioral problems* is larger than the 5% which can be expected on the basis of chance alone. These correlations are shown in Table 6.1.3. There is a slight correlation between information given by the parents and the child's behavioral problems. As one or both parents have given the child more information about the diagnosis and prognosis in the initial stage of the disease, both the mothers and fathers judge their child to be less rebellious. Furthermore, there is less bed-wetting by these children as they have received more information about the diagnosis from their parents in the initial stage of the disease. These relationships are found among children in all age groups. The degree of the child's openness and the degree of the child's eating problems, sleeping problems, and problems at school, are not related to the way the parents gave information about the disease. Partial correlations are not shown in Table 6.1.3 because the child's defensiveness does not appear to influence the relationships.

Table 6.1.3
Pearson correlations (r) between the communication variables "information about the diagnosis" (CSP-ID) and "information about the prognosis" (CSP-IP) on the one hand, and several behavioral problems of children in all age groups, on the other hand.

		Information given by the parents	
Behavioral problems of the child	n	about the diagnosis r	about the prognosis r
Calm versus rebellious behavior, assessed by the mother (BAP-CR)	81	-.24*	-.24*
Calm versus rebellious behavior, assessed by the father (BAP-CR)	78	-.26*	-.25*
Bed-wetting, assessed by the mother (PBAP-B)	81	-.34**	-.17
Bed-wetting, assessed by the father (PBAP-B)	78	-.29*	-.22

* = p<.05
** = p<.01

Information and the child's emotional experience of family relations. The way the parents gave information is not related to the child's emotional experience of family relations.

The emotional experience of family relations in children in all age groups has been measured as the degree of positive and negative feelings which the child experiences towards his or her mother, father, and siblings. We found no significant correlations between the variables information about the diagnosis or prognosis given by one or both parents and the variables referring to how the child experiences the family relations. There is also no relationship if the child's defensiveness is taken into account. This means that the way the parents gave information about the disease is not related to the degree of positive or negative feelings children experience towards their parents and siblings. When relating the feelings the child experiences towards the mother or father to the way the group of mothers or the group of fathers gave information, again no relationship was found between information and the emotional experience of family relations.

Information and the child's positive feelings. The way parents gave information is not related to the child's expression of positive feelings.

Positive feelings have only been measured among the 4 to 12 year old children. These are the positive feelings projected in the hospital play. We found no significant correlations between the variables *information about the diagnosis or prognosis given by one or both parents* and the variable *positive feelings in the child*. This means that the parents' way of giving information is not related to the child's expression of positive feelings.

Communication about the emotional experience and the child's emotional reactions

The children's emotional reactions are not related to the communication of their parents about the emotional experience of the disease.

Communication about the emotional experience is operationalized as actively asking the child how he or she experiences the disease (CSP-CE), as expression of worry (CSP-EW), and expression of grief (CSP-EG) to the child by one or both parents. These communication variables do not appear to be related to the child's various emotional reactions. The number of significant correlations is below the 5% which can be expected on the basis of chance alone. This means that the degree of the child's anxiety and feelings of depression, the degree of the child's positive feelings related to the situation created by the illness, the degree of positive and negative feelings the child experiences towards the parents and siblings, and the extent of the child's behavioral problems according to the parents, all do not have any relationship with the communication style of one or both parents, whether or not they actively inquire how the child experiences the disease and whether or not they express worries or grief to the child. Even if the child's defensiveness has been taken into account, no relationship can be found between these communication variables and the child's emotional reactions. If the communication variables of the group of mothers or the group of fathers are separately related to the feelings which the child experiences towards the mother or father, no relationship can be found between these communication variables and the child's emotional experience of family relations either.

The absence of a relationship between communication about the child's emotional experience and emotional reactions is remarkable because some parents do observe that their behavior on this point could confuse the child. For example, in the interview, a father of a ten year old girls says:

> "At the hospital I was calm the entire day, but when I got home I just kept on crying. I didn't break down in front of her. Once she said to my wife: I never see daddy cry. Doesn't he care? My wife explained that I cried too, but that I preferred to do this when I was alone."

It is questionable if and to what extent parents succeed in hiding their emotions in the presence of the child. The parents may believe they are hiding their worry and grief from the child, while the child actually does perceive the parents' emotions. We quote the father of a five year old girl as an example:

> "When my wife and I couldn't take it anymore, we'd leave the room. I don't think she noticed it...But she did say once: Sometimes I am sad and so are you."

On the other hand, it appears that children find it hard to deal with their parents' grief. A thirteen year old girl relates in the interview:

> "My father and mother have certainly had a shock. They've been very sad. I wasn't really all that sad myself. I don't know...they worry a lot about me and I don't really like that. I don't like it at all that my own parents are so sad about me."

Several times it is apparent in the interviews that children actively attempt to control their parents' and their own emotions. A mother of an eight year old boy relates:

> "When we brought him to the hospital I was actually hysterical. I didn't do anything but cry the first few days. Then he said: Mommy, if you won't cry anymore then I won't cry here anymore either. I'll only cry hard once when I come home. But he never did. That child is so brave, so cheerful. That's why I have to be brave too."

A nine year old boy relates a similar case:

> "When my mother was with me in the hospital she was always crying and that made me cry too. Then I said to her: If you won't cry anymore, then I won't either. And she never cried again. Then she always came in smiling."

More than one-third of the 8 to 16 year old children indicate in the interview that they hide their grief from their parents. There is a slight correlation between the expression of grief by the mother and the concealment of grief by the child ($r=.28$, $p<.05$). If mothers express grief to their child, the child shows a tendency to hide his or her grief. These attempts by the child to control emotions indicate double protection: not only protection of the parents - "it's so difficult for them anyway" - but also self-protection. If the parents break down, the child will too.

Communication about the disease and the child's emotional reactions

Children take the initiative to talk about the disease with their parents more often if it can be inferred from their emotional reactions that they are having a difficult time. They talk more with their parents if they are sad and pessimistic about the outcome of the disease and if they display more behavioral problems (sleeping problems and bed-wetting). If parents take the initiative to discuss the disease with their child relatively often, the older children express less negative expectations for the future and talking about the disease during the interview arouses less anxiety in them. The young children, on the contrary, exhibit more anxiety and tension as parents discuss the disease with them more often. The older children may be less anxious during the interview, but they project more feelings of anxiety and frustration about the disease if their parents talk with them about the disease relatively often. If parents are used to talking freely with others about the disease in the presence of the child, the child displays less sleeping problems, but projects more feelings of frustration. Moreover, the older children project more feelings of anxiety and pessimism about the outcome of the disease.

Finally, the emotional reactions of the child have been studied according to their relationship with the communication variables *communication about the disease at the child's initiative* (CSP-CIC), *communication about the disease at the parents' initiative* (CSP-CIP), and *indirect communication about the disease* (CSP-IC). This involves the frequency of the child and parent discussing the disease in the current stage. Indirect communication refers to the parents speaking or not speaking freely about the disease with others (relatives and friends) in the presence of the child. The number of significant correlations between these communication variables and the variables referring to the child's emotional reactions is greater than the 5% which can be expected on the basis of chance alone. The findings are explained further below.

Communication about the disease at the child's initiative. As children project more feelings of grief and pessimism, they more often take the initiative to talk with one or both parents about the disease in the current stage. The frequency of the children taking the initiative to talk about the disease with one or both parents is also associated with other behavioral problems of the children, i.e. sleeping problems and bed-wetting.

Table 6.1.4
Pearson correlations (r) between the communication variable "communication about the disease at the child's initiative" (CSP-CIC) and several emotional variables of the child.

Emotion variables of the child	Communication about the disease at the child's initiative	
	n	r
Projective measures:		
Grief (HP-G) 4 to 12 year olds	58	.28*
Pessimism (IBC-P) 13 to 16 year olds	24	.52**
Behavioral problems:		
Sleeping problems, assessed by the mother (PBAP-SL) 4 to 16 year olds	81	.35**
Sleeping problems, assessed by the father (PBAP-SL) 4 to 16 year olds	78	.24*
Bed-wetting, assessed by the mother (PBAP-B) 4 to 16 year olds	81	.23*
Bed-wetting, assessed by the father (PBAP-B) 4 to 16 year olds	78	.30**

* = p<.05
** = p<.01

In Table 6.1.4, those emotional variables are included which are significantly related to the variable *communication about the disease at the child's initiative*. The other emotion variables do not correlate significantly with this communication variable. This means that the frequency of the child taking the initiative to talk with the parents about the disease in the current stage does not correlate with anxiety, with how the child experiences family relations, or with the child's positive feelings. The child's defensiveness does not appear to influence the relationships.

Children who are more depressed (more grief and more pessimism) make more attempts to talk about the disease with their parents. This finding only occurs among the projective measures. The direct measures of depression also have a positive relationship with this communication variable, but the relationship is not significant.

Thus children demonstrate a greater need to talk about the disease with their parents if it can be inferred from their emotional reactions that they are having a difficult time. This can be inferred from a stronger display of behavior which indicates emotional problems (sleeping problems and bed-wetting) and from a higher degree of depression (the projection of feelings of grief and pessimism). As we will describe in section 7.8, the communication mainly consists of discussions about the necessity of continuing treatment and/or checkups, about how long a cure will take, and about the possibility that the disease will recur. There are no indications, at least among the 8 to 16 year old children, that the greater need for discussing the disease with the parents is based on a greater need for information about the disease. In anticipation of section 7.3, it can already be mentioned here that the variable *informational needs* of the children is not related to the variable *communication about the disease at the child's initiative*, nor to sleeping problems, bed-wetting, or the projection of feelings of depression. But sleeping problems and bed-wetting occur more often in this age group among children who report finding it hard to obtain information about their disease and to talk about their disease. Moreover, bed-wetting occurs more often among children who report that they have less sources for obtaining information and for talking about their disease. Children who find it hard to talk about their disease and experience that they cannot easily turn to others, appear to attempt talking with their parents about the disease just as often as children who find it somewhat easier to talk about their disease and experience that they can easily turn to others.

The question remains whether children are mainly trying to confide in their parents about their problems and feelings and wish that their parents would share these with them, or whether they are seeking support in order to be able to endure the treatment and are asking for reassurance that they will get better or stay better. For example, a nine year old boy relates in the interview:

"I do talk a lot with my mother: About how long these treatments will have to go on; About what other things they want to do with me; How long it all will take; And whether it will get worse. At the start my mother did know I would get weaker all the time and that it would get worse all the time. But she didn't tell me that. She didn't tell me because she thought: Then he'll get upset. Then my mother said: Don't worry about it too much. We'll see when the time comes. It will be alright. It will turn out alright. I think she's good at telling those kinds of things."

On the one hand, the young boy confides in his mother about his gloomy expectations: "Won't it get worse?" and, on the other hand, he seems satisfied with the reassurance his mother offers him: "I think she's good at telling those kinds of things."

Communication about the disease at the parents' initiative. If parents take the initiative to talk about the disease with their child relatively often, the older children exhibit less negative expectations for the future and less anxiety when talking about the disease during the interview. The younger children, on the contrary, express more anxiety and tension as parents talk to them about the disease more often. The older children may be less anxious during the interview situation, but they project more feelings of anxiety and frustration related to the disease if their parents often talk to them about it.

The communication variable *communication about the disease at the parents' initiative* is significantly correlated with several anxiety and depression variables of the children. These correlations and the partial correlations, from which the effect of the child's defensiveness (8 to 16 year olds) has been removed, are presented in Table 6.1.5.

The direction of the relationship of the direct measure of anxiety (STAIC-Anxiety-state) appears to be the opposite of the projective measures of anxiety. As one or both parents take the initiative to talk about the disease with the child more often, the child reports less anxiety during the interview, but projects more feelings of anxiety and frustration and becomes blocked more often during the hospital play. There is an age effect in the discrepancy between the anxiety-state during the interview and the blocks during the hospital play. Among the group of children between the ages of 4 and 7 years, the correlation between the communication variable *communication about the disease at the parents' initiative* and the number of blocks is positive ($r=.35$), but the correlation among the group of children between the ages of 8 and 12 years is negative ($r=-.22$).

Table 6.1.5
Pearson correlations (r) and partial correlations (part.r) between the communication variable "communication about the disease at the parents' initiative" (CSP-CIP) and several emotion variables of the child.

Emotion variables of the child	Communication about the disease at the parents' initiative			
	n'	n"	r	part.r
Direct measures:				
Anxiety-state (ST-AS) 8 to 16 year olds	56	56	-.30*	-.28*
Negative expectations for the future (NE-f) 8 to 16 year olds	56	56	-.30*	-.27*
Projective measures:				
Blocks (HP) 4 to 12 year olds	58	32	.29*	.25
Anxiety and frustration (IBC-AF) 13 to 16 year olds	24	24	.39	.49*

part.r = correlation between the variables after removing the effect of defensiveness
n' = sample size when calculating the correlations
n" = sample size when calculating the partial correlations
* = p<.05

Thus, among the 8 to 12 year old children, there is no discrepancy between the anxiety-state during the interview and the number of blocks during the hospital play. Both decrease slightly as the parents talk about the disease with the child more often.

It seems that talking about the disease during the interview and during the hospital play arouses less anxiety and tension in children between the ages of 8 and 12 years if they are also more used to talking about it with their parents. However, this does not apply to the younger children (4 to 7 year olds). From the blocks in the hospital play, we can infer that this group exhibits more tension and anxiety as their parents talk about the disease with them more often. For the older children (13 to 16 year olds) no explanation can be found for the discrepancy between the direct measure and the projective measure of anxiety. As parents take the initiative more often to talk about the disease with children in this age group, the children exhibit less anxiety and tension during the interview, but project more feelings of anxiety and frustration. The latter is especially the case if the influence of the child's defensiveness is removed. The discrepancy cannot be explained by an age effect on the anxiety-state scale.

Finally, both the 8 to 12 year olds and the 13 to 16 year olds have less negative expectations for the future as their parents talk to them about the disease more often. The other emotion variables do not correlate significantly with this communication variable. How often the parents take the initiative to talk with the child about the disease in the current stage is thus not related to the way the child experiences the family relations, expresses positive feelings, or displays behavioral problems.

It is possible that the slightly negative relationship between communication about the disease at the parents' initiative and the negative expectations for the future in the child, indicates that parents themselves are more inclined (dare) to discuss the disease when their child is hopeful and confident about the future, but avoid the topic when the child is depressed. It is also possible that this relationship indicates that parents are reasonably good at reassuring their child about the outcome of the disease and at giving the child hope for the future. A correlation cannot give us the answer, but there are indications that the first explanation is most likely. The child's anxiety and depression is rarely a reason for parents to talk with the child about the disease, as will become apparent in section 7.8.

Indirect communication. If parents are used to talking freely with others about the disease in the presence of the child, the children have less sleeping problems but project more feelings of frustration. Furthermore, the older children project more feelings of anxiety and pessimism about the outcome of the disease.

The communication variable *indirect communication* is significantly correlated with several emotion variables of the child. These are presented in Table 6.1.6. Talking freely about the disease by one or both parents with others (relatives and friends) in the presence of the child appears to be associated with more feelings of frustration in the 4 to 12 year old children and with more feelings of anxiety, frustration, and pessimism in the 13 to 16 year old children. It concerns the projection of feelings by the children. The relationships do not appear to be influenced by the child's defensiveness. The relationship between the communication variable *indirect communication* and the direct measures of the child's anxiety

Table 6.1.6
Pearson correlations (r) between the communication variable "indirect communication" (CSP-IC) and several emotion variables of the child.

Emotion variables of the child	n	Indirect communication by the parents r
Projective measures:		
Frustration (HP-F) 4 to 12 year olds	58	.30*
Anxiety and frustration (IBC-AF) 13 to 16 year olds	24	.41*
Pessimism (IBC-P) 13 to 16 year olds	24	.45*
Behavioral problems:		
Sleeping problems, assessed by the mother (PBAP-SL) 4 to 16 year olds	81	-.27*
Sleeping problems, assessed by the father (PBAP-SL) 4 to 16 year olds	78	-.21

* = p<.05

and depression is also positive, but not significant. The indirect communication is not related to the child's experience of family relations or expression of positive feelings. In contrast with this result, we found that freely talking about the disease with others by one or both parents in the presence of the child is associated with less sleeping problems in the children. This relationship is only significant when the mother's assessment of the child's sleeping problems is taken into account.

In the interview, some parents describe situations which clarify the slightly negative relationship between sleeping problems and indirect communication. For example, a mother of a ten year old girl relates:

> "When we have visitors we're careful what we say about her illness as long as she's with us. I don't think it's right

to say everything in front of the child. And luckily most people understand they shouldn't ask too many questions. We can do that when she's in bed. But she often gets out of bed and I notice she's listening at the top of the stairs. Then she's curious what we're all talking about."

The results indicate that children's anxiety, frustration, and feelings of pessimism increase when the children are regularly confronted with their disease through the conversations taking place "above their heads". On the other hand, when parents are careful what they say to others about the disease in the presence of the child, it seems to arouse the child's suspicion.

In the hospital play, there is one scene in which the doctor comes to talk with the parents. Here the children (4 to 12 year olds) are asked: "Where are they going to stand?" Sixty percent of the children spontaneously place the figures (father, mother, and doctor dolls) in the corner of the room or even outside the room. Where the figures are placed does not appear to be related to the indirect communication (talking freely or not freely about the disease with relatives and friends in the presence of the child) nor to the way in which one or both parents talk with the doctor (talking freely or not freely about the disease with the doctor in the presence of the child). In this part of the hospital play children are also asked whether the child (the doll in bed) listens to what the doctor and mommy and daddy are telling each other, and how the child feels about it. More than three-quarters (76%) of the children say that the child listens or tries to listen. This situation appears to arouse curiosity and suspicion, especially in those children who place the figures far away. Characteristic examples are such statements as: "They're being secretive and then he/she thinks: maybe I'm not doing so well?" or "Then he/she is a bit curious and then he/she thinks that the test result isn't so good. But the test result is good."

The ten year old girl, mentioned before, whose mother said she stood at the top of the stairs listening to the conversations of her parents with relatives and friends, places the figures far away and says:

> "She isn't listening because she doesn't think that's very nice. But she feels bad about it. She's a bit worried because the doctor is talking with mommy and daddy. Then she thinks there's something wrong."

A ten year old boy says:

"He doesn't like it. He'd like them to stand closer. I think he's listening very hard. He really wants to know how he's doing. Of course he thinks they're talking about something that he's not allowed to know. He thinks that what the doctor is telling must be very important because he's not allowed to be there."

As far as the youngest children (4 to 7 year olds) can verbalize what the child thinks about the doctor talking with mommy and daddy, they say: "That's o.k., because the doctor says that he/she can go home" or "It's not so good because he/she wants to talk with mommy and daddy and play games."

6.2. The relationship between the communication style and the emotional reactions of the parents

We looked for a possible relationship between the children's emotional reactions and the communication style of one or both parents. The parents' emotional reactions, on the other hand, have been examined as to their relationship with the parent's own style of communication with the child. Because the sex of the parent is slightly related to the communication style and is clearly related to the parents' emotional reactions (see section 8.2), the relationships between the communication variables and emotion variables among the group of mothers and the group of fathers have been determined separately, and have been tested by Pearson correlations. The test results show clear differences in the relationship between communication variables and emotion variables of the mothers and the fathers. The results can be summarized as follows:

- Fathers who have informed their child about the nature and possible implications of the disease at an early stage, experience stronger negative feelings including anxiety, insecurity, and helplessness than fathers who have informed their child later or almost not at all. The emotional reactions of the mothers are not related to the way they informed their child.
- Among the mothers, communication relating to the emotional experiences about the disease is associated with more psychological stress reactions and more feelings of loneliness and isolation, feelings of helplessness, anxiety about not being able to keep it up, and feelings of guilt. No relationship is found among the fathers between this aspect of the communication style and the emotional reactions.
- As the child takes the initiative to talk with the mother about the

disease more often, the mother is more pessimistic about the course of the child's illness. No relationship is found among the fathers between the frequency with which the child takes the initiative to talk with the father about the disease and the father's emotional reactions.
- The frequency of the parents taking the initiative to talk with their child about the disease is not related to the parents' emotional reactions.
- Mothers who freely talk about the disease with others in the presence of the child are less pessimistic about the course of their child's illness. There is no relationship between the fathers' indirect communication and emotional reactions.

On the whole, the relationships we found are not very strong (i.e. the correlations are not high), and do not support our hypothesis that parents who communicate more openly about the disease with their child experience less negative emotional reactions and more positive feelings. An open communication style with the child does not appear to be related to positive feelings in the parents. With regard to some aspects of the communication, an open communication style even appears to be associated with a more negative emotional experience of the situation, by either the fathers or the mothers.

The influence of biographical and disease variables on the communication style and emotional reactions of the parents is described in section 8.2. Whenever these variables correlate either with the communication variables or the emotion variables, this effect has been removed by means of partial correlations. However, they do not appear to influence, in any way, the relationships found between the communication variables and emotion variables of the parents (the partial correlations are almost equal to the correlations).

The emotional reactions of the parents consist of twelve variables. These are the directly measured psychological stress reactions, psychosomatic stress reactions, anxiety-state, use of sleeping pills and sedatives, frequency of visits to the doctor, and pessimism about the course of their child's illness. (The last three variables are considered to be an expression of emotional problems and, as such, are classified as emotional reactions.) The other variables are the projectively measured situation-specific feelings of loneliness and isolation, feelings of anxiety and insecurity, positive feelings, feelings of helplessness, anxiety about not being able to keep it up, and feelings of guilt. The relationships between these emotion variables and the communication variables are presented in three groups. First relating to information about the disease, subsequently relating to the communication about the emotional experience, and finally relating to the communication about the disease. When relevant, qualitative data from the interviews are used to illustrate the quantitative results.

Information and the parents' emotional reactions

Fathers who have given their child more information about the diagnosis and the prognosis in the initial stage of the disease exhibit more negative emotional reactions than fathers who have given their child less information and/or information at a later stage. There is no relationship between the mothers' way of informing their child and the emotional reactions which the mothers experience.

The number of significant correlations among the group of fathers between the communication variables *information about the diagnosis* and *information about the prognosis*, on the one hand, and the emotion variables, on the other hand, is greater than the 5% which can be expected on the basis of chance alone. These correlations are presented in Table 6.2.1, as well as the correlations among the group

Table 6.2.1
Pearson correlations (r) between the communication variables "information about the diagnosis" (CSP-ID) and "information about the prognosis" (CSP-IP), on the one hand, and several emotion variables of the mothers (n=81) and of the fathers (n=78), on the other hand.

	Informing the child			
	about the diagnosis by the		about the prognosis by the	
Emotion variables of the parents	mothers r	fathers r	mothers r	fathers r
Direct measures:				
Use of sleeping pills and sedatives (MC-S)	-.02	.15	-.14	.31**
Pessimism about course of child's illness (PI)	.06	.40**	-.07	-.01
Projective measures:				
Anxiety and insecurity (IBP-AI)	.02	.29**	.20	.27*
Helplessness (IBP-H)	.08	.13	.19	.24*

* = $p<.05$
** = $p<.01$

of mothers which have been included for purposes of comparison. It is striking that the relationships among the group of mothers are found to be entirely different from the relationships found among the group of fathers. On the whole, the correlations are not high so the relationships have to be qualified as weak. They have the following meaning. As the fathers have given more information about the diagnosis to their child in the inital stage of the disease, they are more pessimistic about the course of their child's illness in the current stage and project more feelings of anxiety and insecurity. As the fathers have given more information about the prognosis to their child in the initial stage of the disease, they use sleeping pills and sedatives more often in the current stage of the disease and project more feelings of anxiety and insecurity, and also more feelings of helplessness. The other emotional reactions of the fathers, and their positive feelings too, are not related to the way they informed their child. Among the mothers, no relationship can be found at all between the way they informed their child about the disease and their emotional reactions, either with negative emotional reactions or with positive feelings they experience.

The different results among the mothers and fathers cannot be attributed to a different communication style of mothers or fathers. The extent to which they informed their child about the disease and the time they did so is the same among both groups (see Appendix V and section 7.1 and 8.2). The different results among the mothers and fathers cannot be attributed either to a difference in the use of sleeping pills and sedatives, to a difference in the degree of pessimism about the course of the child's disease, or to a difference in the degree to which feelings of anxiety and insecurity and feelings of helplessness are projected by the group of mothers and the group of fathers (see section 8.1).

Communication about the emotional experience and the parents' emotional reactions

The mothers' communication with the child relating to the emotional experience of the disease is associated with more psychological stress reactions and more feelings of loneliness and isolation, feelings of helplessness, anxiety about not being able to keep it up, and feelings of guilt. Among the fathers, there is no relationship between the communication of the emotional experience of the disease and their emotional reactions.

The three communication variables relating to communication about the emotional experience of the disease involves actively asking the child about worries and grief, and to expressing worry and

Table 6.2.2
Pearson correlations (r) of the communication variables "communication about the child's emotional experience" (CSP-CE), expressing worry (CSP-EW), and expressing grief (CSP-EG) with several emotion variables of the mothers (n=81).

Emotion variables of the mothers	Communication variables		
	Communication about the child's emotional experience r	Expression of worries towards the child r	Expression of grief towards the child r
Direct measures:			
Psychological stress reactions (W-P)	.08	.13	.31**
Projective measures:			
Loneliness and isolation (IBP-LI)	.31**	.12	.08
Helplessness (IBP-H)	.04	-.01	.25*
Anxiety about not being able to keep it up (IBP-AK)	.18	.26*	.17
Feelings of guilt (IBP-G)	.13	.38**	.01

* = p<.05
** = p<.01

grief towards the child. These three communication variables only have a number of significant correlations with the emotion variables of the mothers. This number is greater than the 5% which can be expected on the basis of chance alone. These correlations are presented in Table 6.2.2. Most of the correlations are not very high, but indicate that mothers who actively ask the child how he or she experiences the disease project more feelings of loneliness and isolation; that mothers who express their worries to the child project more anxiety about not being able to keep it up and more feelings of guilt; that mothers who express their grief to the child report more psychological stress reactions and project more feelings of helplessness. Among the group of fathers, the correlations between these communication variables and the emotion variables are not significant except for one. This single significant correlation must be attributed to chance.

Whereas the way the child is informed is only related to the emotional reactions of the fathers, communication about the experiential aspects of the disease is only related to the emotional reactions of the mothers. If they focus more on the child's emotional experience and express more of their own emotions towards the child, they experience more unpleasant emotions. The difference in the relationships found among the mothers and fathers can only be related in one respect to a difference in communication style and emotional reactions. The mothers express grief to their child more often than the fathers (see section 8.2) and they report more psychological stress reactions than the fathers (see section 8.2). If the mothers experience more psychological stress, then perhaps they are less able to control their emotions in front of the child. Another explanation may be that women usually express more emotions, which is not only apparent when completing a questionnaire, but also in their behavior towards the child. Otherwise there are no differences in the communication style and in the projected emotion variables between mothers and fathers which could explain the discrepant results. If it is true that fathers are more reluctant to express their emotional experience of the situation to the child, then this can be illustrated by using a statement made by the father of a ten year old boy. In the interview the father relates:

> "I keep on trying to find out what he's thinking. I think this is important. He himself is convinced he'll get better. Of course I'll get better, he says. I think this is a dilemma. He has a very malignant tumor so I can't be so optimistic myself. On the one hand, you want to be as realistic as possible with him. Try to reduce his optimism a bit. On the other hand, it's also very important to help him bear up. If he would all of a sudden go to the other extreme and would say: I don't believe in it anymore, I don't want to go on, then I'd find that terrible too."

On the one hand, this father's statement expresses the hope that his son will define and perceive the situation in the same way. On the other hand, the father attempts to protect the child from his own feelings of pessimism. Thus the father simultaneously protects himself from the despair which his pessimism would arouse in the child.

Communication about the disease and the parents' emotional reactions

As the child takes the initiative to talk with the mother about the disease more often, the mother is more pessimistic about the course of the child's illness. There is no relationship with other emotional reactions of the mothers, either negative or positive. Among the fathers, no relationship can be found between the frequency the child takes the initiative to talk with the father about the disease and the father's emotional reactions. The frequency the parents themselves take the initiative to talk about the disease with their child is not related to their emotional reactions in any way. Mothers who freely talk about the disease with others in the presence of the child are less pessimistic about the course of their child's illness. There is no relationship with other emotional reactions of the mothers. No relationship can be found between the fathers' indirect communication and emotional reactions.

Though we found no more than two significant correlations among the group of mothers between this group of communication variables and the emotion variables, they exceed the 5% which can be expected on the basis of chance alone. Both significant correlations concern the emotion variable *pessimism about the course of the child's illness*. This variable correlates positively with the communication variable *communication about the disease at the child's initiative* (r=.27, p<.05) and correlates negatively with the communication variable *indirect communication* (r=-.32, p<.01). The correlations are low but imply that as the child takes the initiative more often to talk with the mother about the disease in the current stage, the mother is more pessimistic about the course of the child's illness. It also means that mothers who are used to talking freely with friends and relatives about the disease in the presence of the child are less pessimistic about the course of the child's illness. A mother's statement illustrates this relationship. A relapse has recently been diagnosed in her fourteen year old son.

> "When everything was going alright it was easier. Then you can talk freely in his presence. But now that it's come back, I really don't think I can handle it anymore. Now you know that his chances are much worse. Now the big issue is whether he'll get better. I don't think you should talk about this when he's there. You try to protect him from everything and still be honest. That can be very trying at times."

No relationship can be found among the fathers between this group of communication variables and the emotion variables. Thus, here too, the results are different among mothers and fathers. When talking about the disease, the children address the mother just as often as they address the father, and the degree of pessimism about the course of the child's illness is not different among the mothers or fathers. There is no sex difference either in the indirect communication which could explain the discrepant results among the mothers and fathers.

7. Description of the communication process

The communication variables referred to when testing the hypotheses as the parents' communication style are described in detail in this chapter. We will also present the remaining data of the interviews with the parents and children, dealing with communication about the disease between child and parents, communication within the family, at the hospital, and at home. The following subjects will be dealt with consecutively: the information given by the parents to their child, advice about informing their child given to the parents by hospital staff, the parents' attitude towards informing their child about the disease, questions the child asks the parents about the disease, sources of information, information obstacles, and information needs of the child, other sources of information available to the child, the attempts at information control by the parents, the parents informing the siblings, parents' information-seeking behavior, communication about the emotional experience, communication between child and parents about the death of fellow patients, communication between the two parents, communication between child and parents in the current stage of the disease, the child's knowledge of the disease, and the parents' perception of the child's awareness of the seriousness of the disease. The most significant results which emerge from these data can be summarized as follows:

- Even though most parents have told their child that the disease is serious and that it is a long-lasting illness, almost half of the parents have never used the word "cancer" in front of the child.
- Most doctors and nurses never use the word cancer when they talk to the parents about the child's disease.
- More than two-thirds of the parents have discussed the possibility of dying with their child.
- The attitude of the parents towards informing a child about the

disease corresponds with their actual behavior. In the case of a positive attitude, the first matter of importance is that the child keeps on trusting the parents; in the case of a negative attitude, the accent lies on the burden being too great for a child if you would tell a child everything about the disease.
- More than half of the parents have not discussed with each other what they should tell their child about the disease and many parents are not aware of the information given to the child by their partner.
- For more than half of the children, the parents waited for questions before giving information (cancer, possibility of dying); 40% of the children have explicitly asked: "Am I going to die?"
- When the child asked a direct question, almost a quarter of the parents denied that the disease is a form of cancer and that the child could die of the disease.
- A quarter of the children did not want to ask their parents any questions about the disease in an attempt to protect the parents.
- As the children experience a greater availability of sources of information they are less anxious, less depressed, and have a less negative self-esteem.
- As the children experience more information obstacles, they become more anxious and depressed and have a more negative self-esteem.
- The children do not mention the parents as a source of information as often as the parents themselves do.
- Parents who show more information-seeking behavior themselves have already given their child more information in the initial stage of the disease.
- According to the parents, one-third of the children have received undesirable information about the disease from others. Children at school and in the neighborhood and, to a lesser extent, fellow patients have told the child that he or she has cancer and may die.
- Almost half of the parents have attempted to control the information flow.
- At the hospital, the parents are not given much advice about informing the child. A quarter of the parents have received some advice from doctors and nurses. The type of advice given is highly divergent.
- The siblings have been given considerably less information than the sick child.
- Two-thirds of the parents occasionally ask the child about his or her worries and grief.
- One-third of the children attempt to hide their grief about the illness from the parents.

- Two-thirds of the parents occasionally express their worry and grief to the child and many children are aware of their parents' grief even when the parents try to hide their emotions.
- Almost half of the children spontaneously mention the death of a fellow patient. Parents sometimes erroneously think that the child will not have noticed the death of fellow patients in hospital. In the communication with the child about the death of fellow patients, the parents mainly stress the differences in disease process.
- The initiative to communicate about the disease in the current stage of the disease more often comes from the child than from the parent. The children like to determine themselves how often they talk about it.
- There is a clear relationship between the information the parents have given to the child and the knowledge of the disease exhibited by the child. This knowledge increases with age.
- About one-third of the parents think that the child has no idea of the seriousness of the disease, while almost 90% of the children - even the young children - call the disease bad or serious.

7.1. Information given by the parents to the child

Information about the disease which the parents have given to their child. Table 7.1.1 lists the information which parents have given their child. It concerns the communication variables *information about the diagnosis* (CSP-ID) and *information about the prognosis* (CSP-IP), but the time at which the information was given has not been taken into account. The table shows that in most instances one or both parents have told their child that the disease is bad or serious and that it is a long-lasting illness. Most of the children have been told by one or both parents that they have a tumor or a growth and/or the medical term for the disease has been used, for instance, leukemia, lymphosarcoma, osteosarcoma, Hodgkin's disease, etc.

In more than half of the cases one or both parents have told their child that the disease is a form of cancer. Almost three-quarters of the children have been told by one or both parents about the possibility that the disease may recur. In almost three-quarters of the cases one or both parents have told their child that it is not certain he or she will get better. More than two-thirds of the children have been told by one or both parents that they might die of the disease. The table shows a high degree of correspondence between the information given by the mothers and the information given by the fathers. There are no significant differences. It is re-

Table 7.1.1
Percentage of parents who have informed their child about the diagnosis and prognosis.

	Information about the disease		
	by one or both parents (n=82) %	by the mother (n=81) %	by the father (n=78) %
Informing the child about			
Diagnosis			
Seriousness	98	93	82
Long period of illness	95	79	79
Tumor/Growth/Medical term	83	75	63
Cancer	56	51	40
Possibility of relapse or recurrence	71	59	58
Prognosis			
Possibility of not getting better	73	56	55
Possibility of dying	68	52	50

markable that parents have more often discussed the possibility with their child that he or she may not recover and may die, than they have used the word cancer in front of their child. With more than a quarter of the children (27%), parents have never discussed the possibility of not getting better and/or the possibility of dying, or they have denied this possibility to the child. Towards a larger number of children (44%), the parents have never used the word cancer. We will discuss these findings further below. All the children involved in the study have received at least some information from their parents. For 10% of the children this was limited to information about the seriousness and/or the long period of the illness. In half of the cases this involves children above the age of eight. Parents who have not given much information told their child that "the blood is sick", "that bump does not belong there", or have told their child that he or she "will get medicine to get better".

Information about the disease given by parents to children in different age groups. Table 7.1.2 lists the information given by parents to children in different age groups. With the exception of information about the seriousness and duration of the illness, the information given by the parents to the child about the diagnosis and prognosis clearly increases with age (see section 8.2). The most distinct differ-

Table 7.1.2
Percentage of children in different age groups who have been informed about the disease by one or both parents.

	Age groups		
Information given by one or both parents about the	4-7 years (n=26) %	8-12 years (n=32) %	13-16 years (n=24) %
Diagnosis			
Seriousness	96	97	100
Long period of illness	96	97	92
Tumor/Growth/Medical term	69	88	92
Cancer	23	66	79
Possibility of relapse or recurrence	58	69	88
Prognosis			
Possibility of not getting better	62	72	88
Possibility of dying	54	69	83

ence concerns the information that the disease is a form of cancer. This term has been concealed from more than three-quarters of the youngest age group. With regard to the middle age group, this is the case for one-third of the children, and for one-fifth of the oldest age group.

Information about the disease which the children report they have received from the parents. In the interview, the children between 8 and 16 years were asked what their mother and father had told them about the disease. The children's answers to this question are shown in percentages in table 7.1.3. If we compare these percentages with the percentages in table 7.1.1 and 7.1.2, we see a substantial discrepancy between the information the parents report they have given to the children and the information the children report they have received from the parents. This discrepancy should, to a large extent, be attributed to the difference in measurement methods used for the parents and children. The parents could be asked exactly what kind of information they had or had not given to their child. This was not possible in the case of the children. Here we had to accept whatever knowledge the children indicated they had of the disease. We could not ask direct questions about what kind of information they had or had not received from their

Table 7.1.3
Percentage of children (8-16 years) who indicate having received information about the diagnosis and prognosis from one or both parents (n=56).

Information about the	Information received about the disease from one or both parents %
Diagnosis	
Seriousness	30
Long period of illness	7
Tumor/Growth/Medical term	66
Cancer	46
Possibility of relapse or recurrence	18
Prognosis	
Possibility of not getting better	30
Possibility of dying	27

parents. The interviewer would then be placed in an uncomfortable position and would be forced to give the child information which the parents did not intend the child to have.

In spite of the rather high discrepancy, there is a weak correlation between the amount of information which the parents indicate they have given to the child and the amount of information the children indicate they have received from their parents ($r=.28$, $p<.05$). It must be pointed out that the passing on and reception of information was studied retrospectively, and thus we had to call on the memory of parents and children. However, there are no indications that a distorting influence of memory might play a more significant role for the children than for the parents. We conclude this, for example, from the finding that the factor of the *child's age* and the factor *time since diagnosis* do not influence the discrepancy between passing on information and receiving it. This conclusion is then based on the assumption that a stronger influence of the factor *memory* for children should be mainly found among younger children and among children with a longer period of illness who received information in the more distant past. The discrepancy between the information given by the parents and the information received by the children can be partly attributed to a different interpretation of the situation. The following example clarifies this. The mother of a thirteen year old girl responds to the question whether she has told her daughter that she might die of the disease:

> "When there was talk of her leg having to be amputated she did not want to have it done. Then we had no choice but to tell her that if she didn't have this done, she would die. So we told her that."

The girl herself says in the interview that she knows she has a disease which might be terminal. To the question whether her mother or father told her this, she responds:

> "No, I know you can die of cancer. I have seen it often enough in hospital that children died. My father and mother didn't tell me that."

Parents frequently say they felt forced into discussing the possibility with their child that he or she might die of the disease in order to motivate or convince him or her to undergo treatment. Especially in the case of an amputation, the parents say:

> "You can't say, can you, that the leg has to come off because of some harmless disease?"

The parents interpret the phrase "you must undergo this treatment, otherwise you'll die" as a message that the disease might be terminal. The child might interpret this phrase as the message that treatment guarantees recovery, but not as a message that in spite of treatment death might follow. Other reasons for the discrepancy between passing on and receiving information will come up for discussion below.

The point in time at which the parents have informed their child about the disease. Table 7.1.4 lists at which point in time one or both parents have informed their child about the disease. The table shows that an important part of the information has been given in the initial stage. This refers to the time of the first hospital admission when cancer has been definitely diagnosed and treatment is started. In our study this period consisted of an average of 42 days with a range of 15 to 112 days.

Information on the seriousness and duration of the disease and on the medical term for the disease are generally given to the child in the early stages. When the child is told about the possibility of recurrence of the disease, this is done in the majority of cases when treatment has been completed but the child still frequently has to go to the clinic for checkups. When the prognosis is discussed with the child this mostly takes place in the early stages, but a considerable number of children are not informed about the prognosis until a later stage. Only a few parents give a lack of privacy in hospital as a reason for not informing their child until a later stage. There is no relationship between the point in time at which the children are informed and the child's age. There are no differences between mothers and fathers with respect to the point in time at which they informed their child.

Table 7.1.4
Percentage of children who have been informed about the disease by one or both parents at an early or later stage (n=82).

Informing the child about	Information given about the disease by one or both parents	
	at an early stage %	at a later stage %
Diagnosis		
Seriousness	94	4
Long period of illness	79	16
Tumor/Growth/Medical term	74	9
Cancer	39	17
Possibility of relapse or recurrence	30	41
Prognosis		
Possibility of not getting better	51	22
Possibility of dying	46	22

Consultation between the parents about what information to give to the child. Our sample consists of 5 single parent families and 77 complete families. In less than half of the complete families (44%) the parents have discussed with each other what they should tell their child about the disease. There is hardly any disagreement between the partners about the kind of information they should give to the child. A few couples (4%) disagreed on the amount of information they should give to the child. One couple disagreed on whether they should take the initiative to inform the child or whether they should wait for the child to ask questions.

Parents jointly informing the child. In more than half of the complete families (55%) the parents have jointly given at least part of the information to the child. The parents in the remaining families informed the child on their own, without consulting each other. Most parents appear not to be very well informed about the kind of information given to the child by their partner. Particularly those parents who themselves did not give much information to the child express the opinion that their partner probably gave more information, but they are not certain of this.

Information given to the children of single parent families. The five single parent families participating in our study (four women and one man) have not given their child more or less information about the disease than both parents in the complete families. There is also no difference in the point in time at which these parents informed their child.

How difficult is it for parents to inform their child about the disease? More than half of the parents (58%) thought it a difficult moment when they informed their child about the nature of his/her disease, and the majority of the parents (70%) felt anxiety, tension, and/or grief at that moment. More than half of the parents who experienced these emotions (54%) report they did not show the child these feelings. Control over their own emotions is specifically mentioned by the parents as a problem and some parents were so overwhelmed by their emotions that they were unable to give information. A mother of a 16 year old boy relates:

> "My husband and I wanted to tell him together, but I couldn't. I was too upset. So my husband told him but I was there at the time. Later I asked him: If we hadn't told you then and you would have learned it from another person later, what would you have thought? Then I would've thought you were very mean, he said. From that moment on I've always been honest with him. In time I found it less difficult."

Uncertainty about how the child will react when they inform him or her is also quite often mentioned as a difficulty by parents. A father of a ten year old girl says:

> "You have this feeling of doubt. Am I doing the right thing by telling her all this? She was so optimistic ... then if you say there's a chance she might die ... I was afraid she would lose her courage so I didn't tell her that. In time everything gradually became clear to her. She's seen so much misery around her".

Avoidance of the word cancer by the parents. For many parents the word cancer has a nasty sound and many find it hard to use this term in front of the child. A father of a twelve year old girl explains:

"I said: you have to seriously consider the possibility that it might be a tumor, a malignant growth. Then she said: So you mean I have cancer. I didn't want to use that word, but I said: Yes, that's what it is. It's a very loaded word, isn't it. You try to be more subtle ... but ... you have to say the word or you start beating about the bush."

Parents who have avoided using the term cancer in front of their child argue that their child is still too young to understand the meaning of the word or that the child could not bear the burden of knowing he or she has cancer. The latter argument is especially mentioned by parents who have lost a relative or a personal friend of the family because of cancer. A mother of a twelve year old boy relates:

"My husband died of cancer. One year later it turned out that my son also had it. I can't bear to tell him. I can't do that to him. It would take away all his courage to face life. He did ask: Do I have the same as dad? Am I going to die too? I quickly talked about something else. He has barely recovered from the death of his father ... Formerly there never used to be so much talking. I think they talk too much nowadays."

The parents were also asked whether the doctors, nurses, and other hospital staff ever used the word cancer when talking to them about their child's disease. Almost three-quarters of the parents (73%) report that doctors, nurses, and other staff never use the word cancer in front of them. Two-thirds of the parents (66%) do not use this term in hospital themselves either. Outside the hospital, more than two-thirds of the parents (69%) sometimes use the word cancer when talking to others about their child's disease. They mention that people are often startled by the word. The parents who never used the word cancer (31%) say they do not do this because they find it a "nasty", "terrible", or "rotten" word. One parent says:

"Personally I think they should come up with a new word for cancer."

Advice given to the parents by hospital staff on how to inform the child.

As mentioned previously, there is no clear policy on informing children with cancer at the Children's Oncology Center in Amsterdam.

This also turns out to be the case when we scrutinize the advice the parents report having received from hospital staff. A large majority of the parents (71%) indicate there has been no consultation with hospital staff about what to tell the child about the disease.

Advice from doctors. A limited number of parents (16%) consulted the pediatrician on their own initiative about what to tell their child about the disease. In 13% of the cases the doctors themselves took the initiative. According to the parents, the advice given by the doctors varied considerably. Some parents were advised to be honest with the child and tell him or her everything. Other parents were advised to tell things only at the child's request, and other parents were advised not to talk about cancer or the possibility of dying as this would needlessly alarm the child. From the report of the parents, it becomes clear that the doctor goes along with the parents' point of view when giving advice, and supports their views. Parents who had not yet taken a clear stance with regard to informing their child, allowed themselves to be guided by the doctor's advice to a large extent. No matter what kind of advice they were given, the parents trust the doctor's experience and insight when it comes to informing the child.

Advice from nursing and psychosocial staff. Only 10% of the parents have talked with nursing and/or psychosocial staff about what kind of information they should give their child. Both parents and hospital staff take the initiative just as often for this type of consultation. Here too the advice varies considerably and usually supports the parents' point of view. A small number of parents (12%) have discussed, with hospital staff and/or psychosocial staff, what they should tell their child after a fellow patient died in hospital. Sometimes the parents were advised to discuss this with their child and sometimes they were advised to say that this patient had been transferred to another hospital. A mother of a five year old girl who took this last advice says:

> "She was fully aware that the child next to her had died. That child's condition deteriorated and at a certain moment the curtains were drawn. When they were opened again the girl was gone. The next day she asked me about it and I told her the girl had gone to another hospital. She looked at me as if she wanted to say: tell me another one! It was awful. I will never do that again."

The parents' attitude towards informing the child about the disease

The parents' attitude towards informing the child is reflected in the positive and negative effects the parents expect, if a child would be fully informed about the disease. Two attitude scales have been used to make an inventory of these parental expectations and to examine to what extent the attitudes correspond with the parents' actual behavior. With regard to the latter, Table 7.1.5 presents the correlations between the communication variables *information about the diagnosis* and *information about the prognosis*, on the one hand, and the attitude variables, on the other hand. This table shows there is a clear but not very strong relationship between the attitude of the parents and their actual behavior. As the parents expect more positive effects if a child would be fully informed about the disease, they have already given their child more information about the diagnosis and prognosis in the initial stage of the disease. As the parents expect more negative effects if a child would be fully informed about the disease, they have given their child less information about the diagnosis and prognosis or given it at a later

Table 7.1.5
Pearson correlations (r) between the communication variables "information about the diagnosis" (CSP-ID) and "information about the prognosis" (CSP-IP) on the one hand, and the attitude variables of the mothers (n=81) and fathers (n=78) on the other hand.

Attitude variables of the parents	Informing the child about			
	the diagnosis by the		the prognosis by the	
	mothers r	fathers r	mothers r	fathers r
Positive attitude (PAI)	.18	.25*	.25*	.48**
Negative attitude (NAI)	-.48**	-.30**	-.38**	-.46**

* = $p<.05$
** = $p<.01$

stage of the disease. The relationship between giving information and a negative attitude is somewhat stronger than the relationship between giving information and a positive attitude.

There is a high degree of correspondence between the mothers and fathers with respect to their scores on the attitude scales, that is, their expectations about the effects of fully informing a child about the disease. Therefore the percentages mentioned below (in brackets) refer to the entire group of parents. If we look at the positive effects expected by the parents if one would tell a child everything about his/her illness, almost two-thirds of the parents (64%) indicate that this gives a child a sense of security. Most of the parents feel that a child then understands he/she can trust you (85%), knows that he/she can come to you with all of his/her questions (87%), can accept the illness more easily (75%), and that this strengthens the bond between parent and child (79%). Two-thirds of the parents (67%) believe that a child will not feel so alone and again two-thirds of the parents (67%) believe you have a better understanding of your child's feelings. If we look at the negative effects expected by the parents if one would tell a child everything about his/her illness, then half of the parents (49%) feel this would be too great a burden for a child. About one-third of the parents thinks this would frighten the child (37%), that the child would worry too much (39%), and that this only puts ideas into a child's head (32%). Relatively few parents expect that a child would lose courage (21%), would start resisting treatment (18%), or would never be able to be happy again (13%). From the interview we have supplementary data about the parents' motives to give all or, on the contrary, not all the information about the disease to their child. Besides the above-mentioned positive effects, parents who have given their child all the information also emphasize the child's right to know everything: "It is the child's own body". These parents often believe that their child's trust in them would diminish should they withhold information about the disease. They are convinced that at some stage the child will find out what is going on anyway. That is why they prefer to tell the child themselves. Parents who have given little or not all information about the disease to their child often say this is because their child is still so young. Even parents of adolescents sometimes give this as a reason. These parents either believe that their child would not understand the word cancer, or they believe the child would not be able to bear the knowledge that he or she may have a terminal illness.

Attitude change during the course of the illness. Almost one-fifth of the parents (18%) say that their attitude towards what they should tell their child about the disease has changed during the course of the illness. These parents had not given their child much information at first, but in the course of time they learned to speak more openly about the disease with their child. Many of them give, as a reason for this change, that their child has matured and has begun to understand more due to the experiences associated with the disease. Parents also discovered that their child could handle more, accepted the illness better, and assimilated information better than they had expected. Some of the parents attribute this attitude change to themselves. In the beginning they could not handle the situation, but in the course of time they have become used to it. When cancer is no longer identical to death and hope of a positive outcome increases, it is less difficult for parents to talk about it with their child. One father says:

> "It 's become easier to talk about it because my conception of the word cancer has changed. It's no longer directly linked to death. I've come to understand that cancer doesn't always have to be terminal. I take a less gloomy view of it all."

7.2. Questions which the child asks the parents about the disease

Waiting by the parents for the child's questions. Before informing the child, a considerable number of parents have waited for the child to take the initiative. For more than half of the children (52%) one or both parents said they waited for the child's questions before giving a certain type of information about the disease. In most cases this applies to the information that the disease is a form of cancer and that the child may die of the disease.

Questions parents dread. Almost one-third of the parents (30%) report that in the early stages they dreaded questions the child might ask about the disease. Questions dreaded most were: "What have I got?" "Do I have cancer?" "Will I get better?" "Am I going to die?" "Do I have to have the same treatment as the other children here (in hospital), do I have to have so many needles, will I be that sick too, will I be that bald too?" "How long is it all going to take?"
At the time of the study, there are only a few parents (5%) who say they still dread questions the child might ask them. This refers to such questions as: "Will I get better or am I better?" "Can it (the illness) come back? and "Will I die?"

Questions about the disease which the parents report the child has asked them. In 65% of the families one or both parents indicate that the child has actively attempted to get information about the disease from them. According to the parents, the children did not only ask them questions about the treatment, but also about the nature of the disease. It appears that children who have actively requested information about the disease from their parents, received more information from their parents ($r=.29$, $p<.01$). The child's age has no influence on the questioning behavior. Younger and older children both ask their parents questions. The questions often refer to the prognosis. According to the parents, almost half of the children (48%) asked questions about getting better and dying and 40% of the children explicitly asked: "Am I going to die?" It is a striking finding that this question is already asked quite often by younger children. Of the 4 to 7 year olds, 35% asked this question, of the 8 to 12 year olds, 56%, and of the 13 to 16 year olds, 25%. In the interview, the mother of a four year old girl relates with strong emotions how this question took her by surprise:

> "Half a year after A. became ill she got chicken pox too. That's very critical and I had no idea that such a small child could already understand that. When she came home from the hospital, she sat on the couch, looked wide-eyed at me, and said: Mom, am I going to die? At that moment I was completely at a loss. I quickly said: No, of course not honey, whatever made you think that? I had never expected that such a small child would already know that."

Almost a quarter of the parents (24%) denied the possibility of dying of the disease to the children's question on this. This occurs more frequently when younger children are involved than is the case with older children. To the 4 to 7 year olds, parents denied this possibility in 44% of the cases; to the 8 to 12 year olds, in 17% of the cases; to the 13 to 16 year olds, in 17% of the cases. The parents who admitted the possibility to their child that one can die of the disease mostly reassured their child that the chance was very small that he or she would not make it. They pointed out (usually following the doctor's example) that the course of the illness is unique for each child and emphasized the hopeful aspects of the course of the child's own illness. Apparently the children confronted their parents to a lesser extent with the direct question: "Do I have cancer?" According to the parents, 16% of the children asked this question. This was asked by 28% of the 8 to 12 year old children and by 17% of the 13 to 16 year old children. Not one child in the youngest age group asked this question. To the direct question "Do I have cancer?" parents answered no also relatively often. The parents told almost a quarter (22%) of the 8 to 12 year olds and exactly one-quarter of the 13 to 16 year olds that the disease was not cancer following a direct question from the child. Some parents say their child made it hard for them to give an honest answer. One mother of a thirteen year old boy says:

> "He asked several times: Do I or don't I have cancer? But he always asked this when there was someone else present, the neighbor lady, for example. He probably thought, when there's somebody else here she won't go into this. That's what I think."

A similar method of asking questions is reported by a mother of a nine year old girl:

> "A couple of times she asked: Do I have cancer, Mom? She asked that a few times in the car, when it was full of children I had to take somewhere. I can't explain it to her when there are six other children present. I told her I would explain it to her some other time."

Neither these mothers nor the children came back to the question under more convenient circumstances. Parents indicate the amount of questions does not diminish in time, but the questions change. The mother of a thirteen year old girl says:

> "When she was very ill last year, she'd say each evening: Stay and sit with me for a moment, Mom. Will I get better? I don't think I'll get better. So many die of it. She doesn't ask these questions anymore. Now she asks: If I get it again, what then? She also keeps on asking my husband this to make sure we say the same thing."

Parents who report that their child has never sought any information from them about the nature of the disease (this involves 35% of the children) quite often report:

> "He/she kept on asking why he/she had to go to hospital and why he/she had to have these treatments, but he/she never asked about the disease itself."

These parents do not realize that the child might be trying to get information about the nature of the disease by asking these types of questions. Another kind of indirect questioning by the child to get information about his/her own condition can be manifest in questions about dying or deceased fellow patients. For more than half of the children who have never asked their parents questions about their own illness, the parents do report questions about dying or deceased fellow patients. Some parents mention that it is not by questions, but by the child's behavior that they were forced to be open. This behavior is typified by resistance against continued cooperation regarding treatment. For example, the father of a thirteen year old boy relates:

> "I didn't want to tell him he had cancer because his grandfather and his uncle died of it. But after a few treatments he became very rebellious. He didn't want to continue. Then I had to tell him he had cancer and would die if he didn't undergo treatment. Then he said: I thought so. From then on it's never really been a problem anymore."

Questions about the disease which the children report they have asked their parents. In the interview with the 8 to 16 year olds, 61% of the children report they have sometimes asked their parents about the disease. We found that adolescents (13 to 16 year olds) ask their parents questions about the nature of the disease just as often as the younger children (8 to 12 year olds). A very striking finding is that some children do say they have asked their parents whether they have cancer, but not one child reports having asked explicit questions about dying. This contrasts sharply with the data of the parents. One or both parents of 43% of the children in this category report that the child has asked them: "Am I going to die?" A reason for this difference could be that questions about dying are much more emotionally charged for the parents than for the child. Parents stating that their child asked "Am I going to die?", often give a very detailed description of the situation and of the circumstances in which the child asked this question. The children, on the other hand, more often have a vague recollection of questions they have asked their parents. For example, a number of children report that in the early stages they just let everything happen to them. A thirteen year old girl says:

> "In the beginning it's all very strange. It didn't seem real. You don't really stop and think about it. You only realize later what they are doing and why. That's why I don't think I asked many questions in the beginning. I did later though!"

On the other hand, it is possible that the children asked questions about dying at a time when they were very distressed. The reason for the discrepancy between the children's data and the parents' data could be that children have repressed their memory of questions about dying because it is too painful for themselves and/or for their parents. This can be inferred from the answers the children give, in the interview, to the question: "Have you ever found yourself thinking: I'd like to ask my father or mother something about my illness, but you didn't ask it after all?" More than a quarter (29%) of the children answered this question in the affirmative and for the majority of these children protecting the parents appears to be the most important motive. A twelve year old boy says:

> "Sometimes I just wanted to ask if I might die quickly of it, or something like that. That I would suddenly get very ill and probably die quickly. But I never asked that. I was afraid they would get very sad if I asked that."

A ten year old boy answers:

> "Sometimes I'm afraid that if I ask something, my father or mother will also be frightened by it. So I don't ask it."

A fourteen year old girl puts it as follows:

> "A bit strange really. Some children in hospital ask their parents just about everything. But ... everything I wanted to know I already knew. I found out myself. I ask my parents as little as possible. It's already difficult enough for them. I don't think it's necessary to make it even more difficult for them."

Finally a thirteen year old boy says:

> "I sometimes wonder about the treatment ... about if I didn't have that ... if I would die or something. One night in the hospital I began to bleed a lot. I was really scared then. I never told them about it ... never asked whether I could have died then. I don't know ... but I don't like to ask things like that. I think especially my mother would be frightened."

Besides protecting the parents, the above quotes also show a fear of being confronted with the parents' emotions. A few children (7%) found it hard to ask questions or did not dare to ask questions because they feared the answer they might get from their parents. For example, a nine year old boy says:

> "Sometimes I just want to ask my mother if I'm fine now.

If the medicine is helping me. But then I'm afraid of what my mother might say. Yes ... or no?"

A thirteen year old boy kept a question to himself for a long time:

"I sometimes wanted to ask if I had cancer. As I was lying in hospital in the beginning I already thought I had it ... but I wasn't sure either. I didn't ask for a long time because I was afraid they might say yes. Later though I did ask my father. Then I didn't really mind anymore when he said yes."

7.3. Sources of information, information obstacles, and information needs of the child

The information questionnaire for the 8 to 16 year olds consists of three subscales. The scale *sources of information* investigates to what extent the children believe there are sources of information available to get information about the disease; the scale *information obstacles* examines the difficulty the child experiences in obtaining information about the disease; the scale *information needs* measures to what extent the child wishes to be informed about the disease. The distribution of the scores on the three scales are presented below, as well as the relation of these variables to the communication style of one or both parents and to the emotional reactions of the child.

Availability of sources of information, as experienced by the child. Table 7.3.1 presents the distribution of scores on the sources of information scale.

From the table it appears that most children confirm they have sources in their environment for obtaining information about their illness, and a very high percentage of children state they usually get an honest answer to their questions. Some children do test this though. For example, a twelve year old boy says in the interview:

"I find it easier to ask my parents things than the doctor, but I ask questions anyway. Then I can see what the doctor says and what my parents say and whether it's the same. You can play the funniest tricks on them and then you can see whether they're telling the truth or not. Usually they do say the same thing."

More than a quarter of the children declare they have no one to

Table 7.3.1
Distribution of scores on the scale "sources of information" (IQC-SI) for the 8 to 16 year olds (n=56).

Items	Yes %	No %
If I ask questions about my illness, I usually get an honest answer	95	5
If I have questions about my illness, I always have someone to turn to	86	14
I feel I've been able to ask enough questions about my illness	86	14
I usually ask questions when I want to know something about my illness	82	18
I have someone I can talk to about my illness	73	27

talk to about the disease. This could mean that most children experience less difficulty in getting information about the disease than in communicating about the significance of this information. In section 7.3 we discuss other sources of information for the child, besides their parents.

The scale *sources of information* has a number of significant relationships with the communication variables of the parents and the emotion variables of the child. Children who have received more information about the diagnosis in the early stages of the disease, experience a greater availability of sources of information (see Appendix III). As the child experiences a greater availability of sources of information, the child is less anxious, less depressed, and has a less negative self-esteem. Furthermore, bed-wetting occurs less often among these children (see Appendix III). These findings support the results presented in section 6.1.

Information obstacles as experienced by the child. Table 7.3.2 shows the distribution of scores on the *information obstacles* scale. The table shows that more than one-third of the children say they find it difficult to ask questions about the disease and almost one-third find it difficult to talk about the disease. We already mentioned in section 7.2 that the difficulties the children experience when asking their parents questions about the disease mainly stem from the wish to spare their parents anxiety and grief. We may assume that this wish is mainly based on the child's desire to protect him or herself from a confrontation with the parents' emotions. On the other hand, these difficulties also arise, as it turned out, from the children's desire to protect themselves from alarming information and the emotions evoked by this.

Table 7.3.2
Distribution of scores on the scale "information obstacles" (IQC-IO) for the 8 to 16 year olds (n=56).

Items	Yes %	No %
I find it difficult to ask questions about my illness	39	61
I find it difficult to talk about my illness	30	70

The obstacles to information for the child are not related to the communication style of the parents, but there are some significant relationships with the child's emotional reactions and behavioral problems (see Appendix III). As the child experiences more obstacles to information, he/she is more anxious, more depressed, has a more negative self-esteem, has more sleeping problems, and wets the bed more often. The child also displays more rebellious behavior, according to the father.

The information needs of the child. Table 7.3.3 presents the distribution of scores on the scale *information needs*. It appears that almost two-thirds of the children want to know everything about the disease. Well over one-third of the children declare they want to know as little as possible about the disease. A small number of children (13%) answer both questions "I want to know everything about my illness" and "I want to know as little as possible about my illness" in the negative.

A thirteen year old boy explains this during the interview:

> "What I want to know, I ask about. At least that way you end up knowing what you should. But if you find out too much, that isn't good either. Whatever all the other children in hospital have is none of my business. I don't need to know that."

Table 7.3.3
Distribution of scores on the scale "information needs" (IQC-NI) for the 8 to 16 year olds (n=56).

Items	Yes %	No %
I want to know everything about my illness	64	36
I want to know as little as possibile about my illness	36	64

The same number of children (13%) answered both questions in the affirmative. They want to know everything about their illness and they want to know as little as possible about their illness. This does not necessarily point to any inaccuracy on their part when completing the questionnaire. It can also express ambivalence. A nine year old girl points this out in the interview:

> "It isn't very nice to hear that you have a tumor and that I will die, eh ... that it's terminal. I don't know ... it's not nice either way. It isn't nice if you don't know anything and if you do know, it isn't nice either."

All the 8 to 16 year old children were asked in the interview whether they would have preferred it if the parents and/or doctors had not told them certain things about their illness. None of the children appear to prefer this after all and some children have a very strong opinion about their right to information. A girl of thirteen says:

> "I think you have to know everything. I really think it's mean if a child doesn't get to hear everything. That everything is done behind its back. Thinking up all kinds of poor excuses and telling lies ... no."

It is remarkable that the information needs of the child are not related to the way the parents gave information (see Appendix III). However, there is a significant relationship with some other communication variables. The information needs of the child are greater if parents express their grief to the child and if the parents speak freely about the disease with others in the presence of the child. There is, however, no relationship at all between the information needs of the child and the child's emotional reactions or behavioral problems.

Other sources of information for the child

We explored whether the 8 to 16 year olds had other sources of information besides the parents. The children were asked in the interview what doctors, nursing staff, and psychosocial staff in the hospital had told them about the disease. It was also explored to what extent fellow patients, siblings, friends, classmates, or other children and adults in the home environment acted as sources of information. The parents were asked as well whether their child had received information about the disease from others.

Undesirable information which the child has received from others, according to the parents. The parents of 34% of the children report that their child has received undesirable information about the disease from others. This nearly always involved information that the disease is a form of cancer and/or that you might die of the disease. In these cases the parents did not want their child to find out about this. Major sources of undesirable information are schoolmates and children in the neighborhood and, to a lesser extent, fellow patients, relatives, and acquaintances. Doctors, nursing staff, and other hospital staff are not mentioned by any of the parents as sources of undesirable information.

The doctor and other hospital staff as sources of information

The doctor as an information source. The parents were asked what role the doctor played in informing the child. Almost half of the parents (46%) indicate that the pediatrician at the hospital talked to their child about the disease. However, in most cases this did not take place in the presence of the parents. In these cases the parents sometimes found out from the child and seldom from the doctor what kind of information had been given. Many parents (21%) state they do not know whether the doctor has told their child anything about the disease and 33% of the parents do not think this has happened. In 10% of the cases the pediatrician informed the child in the presence of the parents. According to the parents, in most cases the doctor explained that it was a serious disease, that there was a growth or tumor, or that there were bad cells. The medical term (leukemia, Hodgkin, etc.) was often mentioned as well. The doctor only used the word cancer in one case and in one other case the doctor said it was a disease which could be terminal. When explaining the treatment, the high chances of a cure were emphasized to the child.

The family doctor and the pediatricians who referred the child to the Oncology Center have only played a minor role in informing the child. According to the parents, one family doctor and four pediatricians who sent the child to the center told the child in the parents' presence that the disease was a form of cancer. In two cases the pediatrician commented in pessimistic terms on the chances of a cure when talking to the child. If a doctor informed a child about the disease in the presence of the parent(s), then we regarded this as information also given by the parents. On the communication scales *information about the diagnosis* and *information about the prognosis*, this was scored as information given by the parents.

Besides asking the parents, the 8 to 16 year olds were themselves asked which information they had received from the doctors. Almost two-thirds of the children (64%) state they have received information about their illness from the doctor(s). This information usually refers to the medical term (41%), the term cancer (20%), and the possibility of a recurrence of the disease (25%). A number of children (11%) say that the doctor has also talked to them about the possibility of dying. In only a few cases (5%) did the child declare having heard from the doctor that the disease is a form of cancer, while the parents assume that their child has not been told this. Of all the children who report they have talked to the doctor about the possibility of dying, the parents state they have also talked to their child about this themselves. A quarter of the children (27%) who report they have not received any information about the disease from the doctors, experience this as unpleasant, while the others indicate they would prefer to get their information from their parents. One-third of the children (34%) has actively attempted to get information about the disease from the doctor(s). Questions were asked just as often by the younger children (8 to 12 year olds) as by the older children (13 to 16 year olds). Half of the children who did not ask the doctor questions about the disease say they had wanted to ask questions but were afraid to. This was mostly out of diffidence for the doctor. Some children (5%) state they were afraid of the answer the doctor might give them. The remaining children cannot point out what stopped them from asking the doctor questions.

Nursing, psychosocial, and other hospital staff as sources of information. In the opinion of the parents, other hospital staff do not play a role in informing the child. A limited number of parents (13%) report they know that nursing, psychosocial, or other hospital staff has talked to their child about the disease, but as far as they know these persons have never given any information the child did not already possess. According to the children, these persons are not a source of information either. One-fifth of the 8 to 16 year old children do say though that they have talked with nursing and psychosocial staff about the disease, but this always involved a more detailed explanation of information which the child had already received. In some cases (5%) the death of a fellow patient was discussed with the child and reassurance was given regarding their own prognosis. There are only a few children (5%) who did not like it that nursing staff did not give them information about the disease. These children got the impression that this was taboo: if they had questions about their disease they were constantly told to ask the doctor. Most children (73%) did not seek information from nursing staff. One-fifth of the children (22%) report they did not ask questions because they assumed that nursing staff would not have the knowledge required for answering them.

The parents' views on the independent role played by doctors and other hospital staff in informing the child. The majority of parents (59%) express the opinion that doctors, nursing, and psychosocial staff should ask the parents what they can tell the child about the disease. The other parents hold the opinion that these persons can decide themselves what to tell the child. The parents express their trust in the experience and insight of hospital staff concerning the communication with their child about the disease, or as one father puts it: "They are sensible enough to know exactly what they have to say and how."

Fellow patients as sources of information

A number of children (9%) first learned from fellow patients in hospital that their illness was a form of cancer. This is reported by the parents, as well as the children themselves. Even very young children (5 years old) sometimes ask their parents the meaning of the word cancer because the children on the ward talked about this. A twelve year old girl says:

> "When I was in hospital in Amsterdam, I had not been told yet what was wrong. In the other hospital they did tell me I was very ill, but they didn't exactly know yet what I had. In the hospital in Amsterdam there were two girls of my age and when we were allowed out of bed we would sit together and talk. Then I said: Boy I'm glad I

don't have a malignant growth. Then they said: What makes you think that? Everyone here has a malignant growth. Everybody has cancer here. And you too, otherwise you wouldn't be here. I got really scared then. I ran away and started crying. When my father and mother came the next day I said: Why didn't you tell me? I was angry then. Of course it's not easy to tell your own child it has cancer, but I'm not a child anymore, am I?"

The parents also recount that they had found this situation very unpleasant. The mother of a thirteen year old girl says:

"I felt very bad that she learned from other children that she had cancer. It made me feel like I had failed. I had wanted to tell her myself. Children can be very hard. That's what you think then. Afterwards you realize how wonderful children can be to each other. They really support one another better than parents can do."

A sixteen year old girl relates a similar experience:

"In hospital when they were still trying to find out exactly what I had, a girl in the ward said to me: You have cancer because if you didn't, you wouldn't be here. The next day when I was in the elevator with my mother, she was very agitated. She was nervous and stammering and then I said: Before you try to tell me anything, well you don't have to, because I already know I have cancer. I just blurted it out. Later my mother said she thought the elevator had broken down, that it was falling down at a tremendous speed."

Three-quarters of the children report they have discussed each other's illness with fellow patients. Children who have been told by their parents that they have cancer say significantly more often that children in hospital openly exchange information and talk about cancer than children who have not been told by their parents ($r=.35$, $p<.01$). From this it can be inferred that children who have not been informed by their parents that they have cancer, have probably learned more from their fellow patients than they wish to admit to their parents or to the interviewer.

Siblings as sources of information

According to the parents and to the (8 to 16 year old) children themselves, there is virtually no transfer of information by siblings. According to the parents, one brother told the (sick) child that she might die and one girl says her sister told her she had leukemia.

Sources of information in the home environment

Classmates and children in the neighborhood confront the child even more often than fellow patients with remarks like: "You have cancer" and/or "You are going to die, aren't you?". For 20% of the children one or both parents report these incidents, and in nearly all cases it involves (even young) children who had not (yet) been told by the parents that their illness was a form of cancer and with whom the parents had not (yet) discussed the possibility of dying. Ten percent of the 8 to 16 year olds say that classmates or children in the neighborhood have made the above-mentioned comments about their illness. In some cases such events are reported by the child but not by the parents, so that it can be assumed that the percentage of children who have been informed by classmates or children in the neighborhood may be even higher. For example, a twelve year old boy says:

> "Children at school sometimes said to me: You have cancer, don't you. I always said no then because they had told me it was a polyp. They never told me I had cancer, so then you think you don't. Later you start thinking about it. You start having some doubts. Is it cancer or isn't it cancer? I sometimes thought to myself: Should I ask now? But then they might think I'm being a bother and just say the same thing all over again, that it's a polyp."

This boy has clearly been confused by his classmate's remarks. He does not ask his parents for an explanation because he thinks they will deny it. He might even prefer to avoid confirmation of his suspicions for now, so he can keep denying that the disease is a form of cancer.

Many children who know they have cancer say in the interview that the swear word "cancerous bastard", which they formerly used themselves, now has a completely new meaning for them and they get very angry now when other children casually use this swear word. A fourteen year old boy says:

"Some boys in the class always say "cancer" or "cancerous bastard" when they are angry about something. I get really hopping mad then. Then I think, you don't know what you're talking about but I have had cancer. Then I say: You have no idea what you're talking about."

Relatives, acquaintances, and neighbors are also mentioned by 7% of the parents as sources of undesirable information for their child. These people let it slip out in front of the child that it has cancer or might die from it, without the child having been informed about this. Besides this, a large number of parents (55%) indicate that the child has probably talked with more people about the disease, but they are not sure if these people had given any information and, if so, what kind of information was given, as the child has been very tight-lipped about this.

7.4. The parents' attempts at information control

A small number of parents (16%) are sometimes worried that their child might receive undesirable information about the disease from others. For 46% of the children, the parents have attempted to control the flow of information.

Attempts at information control within the family. In 30% of the families the parents have urgently requested the siblings not to pass on certain facts about the disease to their sick brother or sister. This usually relates to information that the disease is a form of cancer and/or the brother or sister might die. In a few cases the parents asked the siblings to keep it a secret that the disease has spread or that the disease might recur again. Also, the parents quite often forbid the siblings to give information to others outside the family. In a quarter of the families they have been asked not to "blab it around" that their brother or sister has a serious disease, has leukemia, has cancer and/or is bald, and wears a wig. In 9% of the families the parents have advised the siblings not to talk about the disease at all with children or adults outside the family. Sometimes the parents also advised the sick child to be careful about what he or she tells the outside world about the disease. Eight percent of the children were advised by the parents not to tell everything to just anybody, because others may only be hungry for sensation and the sick child might be teased about it. The parents of some children (10%) hid newspapers, magazines, or books with information about cancer to prevent their child from taking note of this, and the parents of 16% of the children make sure the child does not see television programs about cancer.

Attempts at controlling information in the family's social environment. The parents of 29% of the families have requested the social environment to keep certain kinds of information about the disease from the child. The parents urgently requested relatives, acquaintances, and teachers not to talk about cancer and/or the possibility of dying in front of the sick child. One father monitored the information which classmates might have given to his fourteen year old son:

> "In the beginning all his classmates sent him a note. I checked all of them. There was one note that said: I heard you have cancer. I made sure he didn't get that one."

In a number of families (7%) the parents requested certain people not to say anything at all to the child about the disease. One mother tried to achieve this at school:

> "I talked to the School Principal. The children are not allowed to talk about my daughter's disease anymore, by order of the Principal."

Attempts at information control directed at doctors and other hospital staff. In a few cases the parents have also requested hospital staff not to inform the child about certain facts of the disease. The parents of 7% of the children have asked the doctor(s) not to use the term cancer in front of the child and not to bring up the subject of the possibility of dying. The parents of 5% of the children urgently requested nursing and psychosocial staff not to inform their child about the death of a fellow patient. The opposite is sometimes the case (5%) when parents urged doctors and hospital staff to give their child all the information and to answer the child's questions honestly. These parents feel it is important that hospital staff follow the same line of conduct as the parents themselves.

7.5. Informing the siblings about the disease

Information about the disease which the parents have given to the siblings. In 10% of the families participating in our study, the sick child is an only child. In well over half of the families (52%) the child with cancer has one brother or sister, and 38% of the families have three or more children (see Appendix I). In those cases where

Table 7.5.1
Percentage of siblings and percentage of sick children who have been informed about the diagnosis and prognosis by one or both parents.

Information about the	Information about the disease given	
	to the siblings (n=64) %	to the sick child (n=82) %
Diagnosis		
Seriousness	92	98
Long period of illness	47	95
Tumor/Growth/Medical term	39	83
Cancer	53	56
Possibility of relapse or recurrence	6	71
Prognosis		
Possibility of not getting better	52	73
Possibility of dying	48	68

one or more of the siblings were 4 years or older (n=62), the parents were asked what information they had given to the siblings about the sick child's disease. Table 7.5.1 shows what kind of information the parents gave to the siblings. For comparison purposes, the information given by the parents to the sick child is also shown.

The siblings have received considerably less information about the disease from their parents than the sick child. They received less information in particular about the long period of illness, about the medical term for the disease, and about the possibility that the sick child's disease might recur. In most of the families the parents did mention that the brother or sister has a serious disease. Many parents report they felt forced to do so because of the reactions of the children to their altered life-style. For example, a father says:

> "She (the other child) could not sleep for quite awhile. She would lie in her bed at night crying. She was also jealous of the attention that her sister received. Then we told her how ill her sister was and then it became clear that she had not been able to sleep because she was afraid her sister would die."

How difficult is it for parents to inform the siblings about the disease? Many of the parents (43% of the mothers and 34% of the fathers) found it difficult to inform the siblings about the sick child's disease. The parents say the greatest problem was the emotions this arouses in them and the need they feel to choose their words carefully so they can pass on information intelligibly and tactfully.

Questions which the parents dread. Only a few parents (6%) have dreaded the questions which the siblings might ask about the sick child's disease. Whenever questions were dreaded, this related to the question whether the brother or sister had cancer and whether he/she would die.

The point in time at which the parents informed the siblings about the disease. Even more so than in the case of the sick child, the parents have given information to the siblings about the diagnosis and prognosis mainly in the initial stage of the disease. Only 9% of the children received additional information from the parents at a later stage.

Questions about the disease which the siblings have asked the parents. Although less information about the sick child's disease has been given to the siblings by the parents, the siblings make just as many attempts to obtain information. In 70% of the families, one or both parents indicate that the siblings have asked them questions (for the sick child this percentage is 65%). An important proportion of the questions (41%) refer to the prognosis. In 30% of the families, the children asked their parents explicitly whether their brother or sister was going to die. The question whether the sick child has cancer was asked by 13% of the children, and the same percentage asked the parents what causes the disease and whether they might get it too. Just like the sick child, the siblings receive more information from their parents if they actively ask for information ($r=.25$, $p<.05$). However this does not mean that all children obtain the information requested from their parents. When children ask whether their brother or sister has cancer, this is denied by parents in more than one-third (38%) of the cases. Almost the same percentage (37%) of parents gave a negative reply to the question whether the brother or sister may die. Among parents who deny to the siblings that the disease is a form of cancer or deny that the sick child might die, there is no corresponding behavior towards the sick child. In most cases (60%) these parents have told the sick child the disease is a form of cancer or he or she might die of the disease.

Information the sick child has given to the siblings. A quarter of the 8 to 16 year old children with cancer (26%) report in the interview that they have told their brother or sister something about their illness. The information which they have passed on is almost exclusively related to the nature of the treatment (needles, infusions, and radiotherapy) or to their experiences in hospital. Only two children say they have given information about the disease itself. One boy told his brother that he had cancer and another boy told his sister that his disease is called Hodgkin's disease.

Undesirable information which the siblings have received. One-fifth of the parents report it has happened that siblings received information from others which the parents consider to be unsuitable. In most cases it concerns statements from schoolmates and neighbor's children who said: "Your brother (sister) has cancer and will die." In one case a child had to face the remark from a classmate that his brother's arms would be amputated.

7.6. The parents' information-seeking behavior and their evaluation of information given by the doctor

The parents' information-seeking behavior. The scores on the scale *information-seeking behavior* (ISP) give an idea of the extent to which the parents seek information about cancer in newspapers, journals, books, and television programs, and the extent to which the parents actively attempt to obtain information about their child's disease from doctors. Some examples of questions from the information-seeking scale are presented in Table 7.6.1. Because the answers from the group of mothers correspond highly with the answers from the group of fathers, the percentages concern the entire group of parents. Most parents do not appear to avoid the information about cancer which they happen to come across, but the number of parents who actively seek information is clearly smaller. Most of the information is obtained from newspapers and women's magazines and to a lesser extent from weeklies, medical journals, and medical encyclopedias. A few parents (14%) have read books which relate the experiences of other parents of children with cancer. The reasons mentioned by parents for reading about cancer are: the need to know more, to get some grip on the situation, to be able to make comparisons, to keep up-to-date with new developments, and to learn what is yet to come. Many parents indicate their involvement with this topic has become much greater since their child's illness. Some parents find the information frightening. They become distressed by all the misery and feel helpless. For this

Table 7.6.1
Percentage of parents who actively seek information (n=159).

Descriptions of information-seeking behavior	%
Sometimes buys books or magazines which contain articles about cancer	37
If one comes across something about cancer in a newspaper or magazine, one usually reads this	88
Goes to the library or a public information center to learn more about cancer	10
Usually watches TV programs about cancer	62
Talks in the hospital to the doctor on duty when one has questions to ask	82
Talks in the hospital to the pediatrician when one has questions to ask	60
Telephones the pediatrician from home when one has questions to ask	56
Reads the instructional information sheets included with the child's medicine	56
Asks the doctor about test results	82

reason, a small number of parents (12%) do not wish to be confronted with this topic at all.

The parents' information-seeking behavior shows a number of significant relationships with the communication style towards the child, especially among the fathers (see Appendix IV). As the parents (mothers and fathers) seek more information themselves, they have given their child more information about the diagnosis at an early stage. Furthermore, the fathers have given more information about the prognosis to the child at an early stage, express their worries to the child, and take the initiative more often to talk with their child about the disease, as they themselves show more information-seeking behavior. These relationships are not found among the mothers. Differences also occur between mothers and fathers if we look at the relationship between the information-seeking behavior and the emotional reactions. There are no significant relationships except a few among the fathers (see Appendix IV). As the fathers show more information-seeking behavior, they are more pessimistic about the course of their child's illness and project more feelings of anxiety and insecurity. To what extent the fathers' information-seeking behavior is an attempt to reduce the existing feelings of pessimism, anxiety, and insecurity, or to what extent it actually leads to an intensification of these feelings, cannot be determined.

Evaluation of information given by the pediatrician. The larger proportion of parents (89%) feel their child's pediatrician has given them sufficient information about their child's disease and appreciate the way this information has been given. But many parents do note that they have to actively ask for information before receiving it. In Table 7.6.1 we see that parents do not always do this. Almost half of the parents adopt a rather passive attitude towards questions they would like to ask the pediatrician. It seems that the doctor is influenced by the parents' attitude, not only concerning advice about informing the child but also when informing the parents. Many parents point out that the tenor of the information they receive from the doctor is very optimistic. On the one hand, this optimism stimulates feelings of hope in the parents, but on the other hand, this could end up contrasting with reality. One father expresses this as follows:

> "In the beginning you cling to the doctor's optimism. But when you see children dying in hospital, you realize it can also come to a bad end and you wonder if that aspect should not be emphasized as well. But well, if you look at it from the doctor's point of view, perhaps it's logical. He has to do his job with complete conviction."

Almost one-third of the parents (31%) point out the difficulty of talking freely with the doctor in the presence of their child. This is especially the case during treatment at the clinic or checkups. The topics the parents do not wish to discuss with their doctor in the presence of the child almost always relate to the child's survival chances. For example, a father of a ten year old boy says:

> "I'd like to ask about his chances, about survival rate, but I don't do that when he's in the room. I think it's o.k. for him to believe that the worst trouble is behind him. What's more, the questions don't help anyway because you know it's only a statistic."

A few parents (9%) sometimes send their child to the waiting room in order to ask the doctor some questions.

Table 7.7.1
Distribution of the item scores of the communication variables "communication about the child's emotional experience" (CSP-CE), "expression of worry" (CSP-EW), and "expression of grief" (CSP-EG) by the parents.

Communication variables	One or both parents (n=82) %	Mothers (n=81) %	Fathers (n=78) %
Sometimes asks whether the child is sad	68	63	58
Sometimes asks whether the child is worried	64	58	53
Sometimes expresses worry to the child	67	62	53
Sometimes expresses grief to the child	73	72	37

7.7. Communication about the emotional experience

Communication about the child's emotional experience and the parents' expressions of worry and grief

Three communication variables of the parents are included in communication about the emotional experience: verbal communication about the child's experience and non-verbal communication, that is, the expression of worry, and expression of grief to the child. The distribution of the item scores of these communication variables is presented in Table 7.7.1.

In the table we can see that in about two-thirds of the cases, one or both parents sometimes ask their child about his or her worries and grief. There is no difference here between the group of mothers and the group of fathers. Parents who never inquire about the child's worries and grief state that they see no reason for this, or find questions superfluous because the child's behavior speaks for itself, or the parents refrain from asking questions because the child always reacts with a rejection or always denies worries and grief. We will return to this in section 8.1. In the case of two-thirds of the children, one or both parents sometimes show their worry about the disease and to almost three-quarters of the children, one or both parents sometimes show their grief. The number of mothers who express their grief to the child is larger than the number of fathers (see section 8.2). There is no difference between the group of mothers and the group of fathers with regard to expressing worries. Most of the parents who sometimes cry in front of the child, explain to their child that his or her illness is the cause. More than a quarter of the parents (28%), however, do not give their child an explanation or deny to the child that his or her illness is the cause. Some parents even deny their grief. One mother says:

> "When it happened once he said: Mommy, are you crying? No dear, I have a cold, I said."

Parents who do not express their worries and/or grief to their child generally give the reason that they do not want to burden or discourage their child. In section 6.1. we already asked the question to what extent the parents succeed in hiding their emotions from the child. The results of the hospital play confirm our doubts. A very high percentage of children project feelings of grief onto the mother and father. In this play, 87% of the children say once or many times that the mother is sad and 84% say that the father is sad. The statements of the younger children (4-7 years) about these emotions of parents do not differ from the older children's statements (8-12 years). As a reason for the parents' grief, it is usually mentioned that the mother and father miss the child, because the child is sick and has to have so many needles. In some cases (16%) children refer to a fatal outcome of the disease, but in most cases this happens in a vague manner such as: "They are sad because they're afraid that something awful will happen to the child" or "When the doctor thinks the very worst." Only two children explicitly state that the parents are sad because their child might die. The separation between parent and child is a source of grief for many children and, according to the children, for the parents. A four year old boy says:

> "Mommy has to cry because he has to stay in hospital so long. Then Mommy not even knows my name anymore."

A four year old girl who says the parents are not sad gives the reason:

> "Mommies and Daddies can't cry at all."

Description of the communication process 169

In the interview, the 8 to 16 year old children were asked whether they noticed their parents' grief and nervousness in the initial stage of their illness. A quarter of the children clearly perceived that their parents were sad. During the first stay in hospital nervousness was noticed more in the mothers (38%) than in the fathers (23%). The parents' attempts to be as cheerful and normal as possible is noticed by the children. An eleven year old girl relates:

> "Well now, I could see I was very ill because Mommy and Daddy would come in with very red eyes. They were very cheerful though, but if they had to cry again they left the room. Just to smoke a cigarette."

The children have also been asked to what extent they express their own grief to the parents. As already mentioned in section 6.1, more than one-third of the children (36%) try to hide their grief from the parents and the children are inclined to do this even more if the mother expresses her grief to the child. There is no difference between the younger (8-12 years) and older children (13-16 years) in perceiving the parents' emotions and hiding their own emotions. The children were asked why they hide their grief from their parents and it appears that the main reason is to protect their parents. They want to prevent their parents from crying and we may assume they want to protect themselves from confrontation with the parents' emotions. In the hospital play it was also examined whether the children perceive emotions of grief in other adults, in the doctor, and the nurse. According to 37% of the children, the doctor is sometimes sad and according to 46% of the children, the nurse is sometimes sad. These percentages are almost equal for the younger children (4-7 years) and the older children (8-12 years). An eleven year old boy relates:

> "If the doctor knows beforehand that he (the child) will not make it, then he'll surely feel sad. Then he'll think about how he must tell the parents. Should he tell them right away or, umm ... should he tell them later after it has already happened."

The same boy says about the nurse:

> "She won't show it if he (the child) is there but afterwards she's very sad because he's so sick. She's just sad because she's not allowed to tell him. That the boy ... that the boy didn't know anything. She's also sad when some

patients have been very nice and, umm...then they die. Then she's very sad."

Some children mention the emotion control of doctors and nurses. They state the doctor and nurse might be sad sometimes, but will not show it. Other children assume that an emotion such as grief is not felt by doctors and nurses because there are so many patients that they get used to it, or because they wanted to work in a hospital themselves and thus cannot be sad. A ten year old boy gives a surprisingly nuanced description of the doctor's emotions:

"I don't think the doctor is really sad. But I think that when a child dies, he feels a bit guilty. But I think on the other hand he also thinks, well, I've done my best, but it didn't work. It's his job. At least I don't think it's unusual for him if a child dies."

Communication about the emotional experience with the spouse

In the interview the parents have been asked their opinion on the frequency and quality of communication with the partner. They have been asked how often they discuss their worries about the illness of their child with their partner in the current stage of the disease, whether they think the frequency is sufficient or insufficient, and whether they are satisfied or dissatisfied with the quality of the communication with their partner. The answers from the group of mothers and the group of fathers show a high degree of correspondence. Well over half of the parents (56% of the mothers and 55% of the fathers) indicate that they talk at least once a week with the partner about the worries concerning their child's illness. Most of the parents (83% of the mothers and 89% of the fathers) hold the opinion that they talk enough with the partner; the remaining parents feel they do not talk enough with their partner. Most parents find the quality of communication with the partner quite satisfactory. Some mothers (17%) and fathers (16%) express dissatisfaction with the quality of communication with their partner about the worries concerning their child's illness. One father comments on this situation:

"My wife deals with this differently than I do. I want to talk about it often. But she doesn't. I need people around me. She doesn't. We often drive to Amsterdam in silence; go the whole way without saying anything to each other. We aren't able to help each other with emotional problems because we cope so differently. That causes tension. It's changing our marriage."

Communication about the emotional experience with fellow-sufferers

The parent discussion groups, organized in the Emma Kinder Ziekenhuis in order to give parents of children with cancer the opportunity to discuss worries about their child's illness with fellow-sufferers, have been attended by almost one-quarter of the parents in our study group (21% of the mothers and 23% of the fathers). Outside the discussion group, 46% of the mothers and 38% of the fathers do have contact once in a while with other parents of children with cancer. The mothers are more positive about this type of contact than the fathers. Seventy-one percent of the mothers express their satisfaction with the communication about their own worries with fellow-sufferers. Among the fathers this percentage is 57. In contacts with other parents of children with cancer, especially the shared experience and the understanding which stems from this are seen as positive. Parents who experience contact with fellow-sufferers as negative or who avoid this contact often give the reason that they have already had enough misery as it is. A mother expresses her negative evaluation in the following way:

"In the parent's room at the hospital nothing else but the children is discussed. Once there was a father who wanted to do something else for a change. He told a joke and I began to laugh. Then some of the parents became very angry. How did we dare to laugh! I got the impression I had to be ashamed."

Communication between the child and parents about the death of fellow patients

Most of the parents (84%) have experienced the death of a fellow patient of their child once or several times. One-third of these parents declare their belief that their child has not noticed any of these events. This belief does not always correspond with the child's report about this. In the interview and/or in the hospital play, 44% of the children spontaneously report events concerning the death of one or several children during their stay in hospital. More than one-fifth of all the children mention they have experienced such a situation, while their parents hold the opinion that this situation either did not occur or their child had not noticed anything. Almost three-quarters of the parents who realized their child noticed the death of a fellow patient, have discussed this with their child and acknowledged the event. Most parents emphasized to their child the differences in disease process. The mother of a twelve year old boy relates:

> "Many children died while he was in hospital. In most cases, it wasn't so difficult to talk about this with him. They had a very different type of cancer. But when one boy died it was difficult. He was just as old and he also had a tumor in his leg and had also had an amputation. This boy had comforted J. when he heard that his leg would have to be removed and showed J. his prosthesis. When this boy died we had to make it very clear to J. that each case is different and that you can't compare cases, because he was comparing himself with this boy and was very depressed about the whole thing."

Some parents, having noticed that their child was aware of the death of a fellow patient, denied this in front of the child by saying this child had gone home or had been transferred to another hospital. Some parents could not talk about this at all with their child. A mother of a ten year old boy says:

> "When he was getting treatment he always shared his room with the same boy. They were always admitted at the same time and the boy became a close friend. But one day that boy was taken out of the room and then died. S. asked about him but I couldn't tell him. He kept on asking, he was aware of things, and he said: But Mom, I really believe he's not alive anymore. Inside I was hoping: Please don't ask me anything else, don't ask me anything, because I can't give you an answer. I had the feeling: if he finds out he will get worse and will die himself."

Some parents expressed their surprise at the children noticing everything, no matter how carefully the hospital staff treat the death of a fellow patient. This is even the case among very young children, as can be seen from what a father relates about his five year old son:

> "He said once: Hey Dad, did you know that children die here? I said: Yes. He said: Why didn't you tell me sooner? Then I said: I didn't think you would understand. He said: Oh but I understand that alright, Dad."

Many parents are amazed at the realistic way the children accept the death of a fellow patient. The mother of a thirteen year old girl says:

> "We have received quite a few death announcements. In the beginning she was upset but now she often just says: Yes, it's awful. Then I say: But doesn't it make you sad? She says: Yes, but Mom, if you won't get well anyway, why should you have to keep on having treatments. Don't think that's any fun either."

When fellow patients have become friends of the child, their death is naturally very difficult to deal with. A sixteen year old girl recounts:

> "Three boys I knew well have died of it. One was, well, my boyfriend. I just couldn't believe it. I still can't. Everytime I go to the hospital, I think he'll just be sitting there. It's really strange, but you just can't accept it."

A number of children and parents point out that for this reason the doctor had not admitted children who were becoming friends for treatments at the same time, in order to discourage the development of close friendships. Both the children and parents completely disagree with this policy. They feel that the friendships are more important than the grief should a friend die.

7.8. Communication about the disease in the current stage of the disease

Communication about the disease between parents and child at the child's initiative

The parents have indicated how often their child has taken the initiative to talk with them about the disease during the month prior to the interview. The distribution of the scores of this communication variable is shown in Table 7.8.1. In this table we can see that almost half of the children turn to one or both parents to talk about the disease once or several times a week. The frequency of the child's taking the initiative to communicate about the disease depends on a number of disease characteristics and the child's age (see section 8.2). Children take the initiative more often to talk with one or both parents when they have been diagnosed recently, when they are still undergoing treatment and have to go to the clinic often for treatment and/or checkups, and when they are reminded of

Table 7.8.1
Distribution of scores on the communication variable "communication about the disease at the child's initiative" (CSP-CIC).

Frequency of communication about the disease at the child's initiative	One or both parents (n=82) %	Mothers (n=81) %	Fathers (n=78) %
Several times a week	20	14	7
Once a week	26	19	16
Less than once a week	27	29	24
Less than once a month	27	39	54

their illness by their physical condition and appearance. Furthermore, young children take the initiative to talk with their parents about their illness more often than older children do. The children do not turn to the mother significantly more often than to the father.

The communication mainly consists of discussions about the necessity to continue treatment and to undergo painful procedures (bone marrow aspirations, lumbar punctures). The communication is also quite often directed at the question how much longer it will take before the child is well and at the possibility that the disease will recur. A mother of an eleven year old girl gives an example:

> "M. has been very down this past week. She still has to have two cycles of chemotherapy and she's dreading it. What if I'm still not better after the last treatment? I wish I was dead, she says. I still try to give her courage. I told her a joke about a burglar who had to climb ten walls and at the eighth wall said he didn't want to go any further. You're such a long way already and then you start saying you don't want to go on with the treatments. Then you're just like the burglar. So I always keep on trying to give her courage."

Communication about the disease between parents and child at the parent's initiative

The parents also indicated how often they have taken the initiative to talk about the disease with the child during the month prior to the interview. The distribution of scores of this communication variable is presented in Table 7.8.2. In the table we can see that

Table 7.8.2
Distribution of scores on the communication variable "communication about the disease at the parent's initiative" (CSP-CIP).

Frequency of communication about the disease at the parent's initiative	One or both parents (n=82) %	Mothers (n=81) %	Fathers (n=78) %
Several times a week	16	10	8
Once a week	15	9	12
Less than once a week	22	18	13
Less than once a month	48	64	67

the parents take the initiative less often than the child itself. There is no difference here between the group of mothers and the group of fathers.

The same disease characteristics which influence the frequency with which the child takes the initiative to talk about the disease also influence the frequency with which the parents take the initiative (see section 8.2). Furthermore, parents of younger children take the initiative more often than parents of older children. Whenever the parents talk to the child about the disease, the main topics of conversation are also the necessity of continuing treatment and the burden and restriction which the child experiences from this. The child's anxiety and/or depressive behavior is the reason for 9% of the parents to talk about the disease with the child. In almost half of the families (48%) neither parent took the initiative to talk about the disease with their child during the month prior to the interview. These parents indicate they do not want to burden the child with their own worries and anxieties or they give the reason that the child does not want to be reminded of the illness. From the interview data of the 8 to 16 year old children, it emerges that the parents adequately evaluate their child's need for communication about the disease. The children indicate a high degree of satisfaction with the frequency of talking about the illness with their parents in the current stage of the disease. Only two children would like to talk more often with their parents and one child feels his parents talk too much with him about this. The majority of the children indicate either that they talk enough with the parents about the disease or they do not mind that they have not talked about it lately. A sixteen year old girl says:

> "When I feel like talking about it, then I'll start the conversation myself. If they (the parents) start to talk about it and

I don't feel like it, I tell them: Let's not bring that up again."

Another sixteen year old girl says:

"I think I talk enough about it with my parents. I decide myself how often I want to talk about it. If I start talking about something else, they stop of their own accord."

The children who report they have not talked with their parents about the disease lately (36%) say they like it this way because they do not always want to think about it. A twelve year old boy says:

"I'd like to forget it as soon as possible because it isn't a nice thing to be reminded of."

The child's communication with siblings and peers

In the interview, the 8 to 16 year old children have been asked whether they sometimes talk about their illness with their brothers or sisters and with friends. It is a striking finding that more than half of the children (58%) report that they never talk with their brothers or sisters about the illness. They mostly mention, as a reason for not talking, that the brothers or sisters "don't understand anyway". Even for the children who sometimes talk about the illness with their brothers and sisters, well over one-third (37%) say that a really good talk is not possible. A lack of knowledge and understanding by siblings is often given as a reason for a negative evaluation of this communication. Nevertheless, it cannot be proven that the way they were informed plays a role here. The way the siblings have been informed by the parents about the disease is neither related to the communication between the sick child and the siblings nor to the child's appreciation of this. Neither is it related to the way the child with cancer has been informed. Half of the children sometimes discuss the illness with friends. The other half never do. Here they also state that the reason for not talking is the lack of understanding for their situation. One-third of the children who sometimes discuss their illness with friends do not evaluate these conversations positively.

Indirect communication

The communication variable *indirect communication* refers to the question whether parents talk freely or not about the disease with relatives and friends in the presence of the child. In 71% of the families, one or both parents speak freely about the disease with relatives and friends in the presence of the child. Among the group of mothers this is 62% and among the group of fathers this is 61%. Many parents remark that speaking freely with others has been made possible by a favorable course of their child's illness. However, there is no clear relationship between a poor prognosis and being reserved when communicating with others (see section 8.2). Neither are there indications that parents wishing to protect their child from certain kinds of information, i.e. that the disease is a form of cancer or that the child might die of the disease, are more reserved when communicating with others. The wish to protect the child from confrontation with the parents' anxieties and insecurities is in most cases mentioned as a reason for not speaking freely with relatives and friends in the presence of the child. Thus the parents are mainly reserved when discussing the chances of a cure and the child's prospects.

7.9. The child's knowledge of the disease

The child's knowledge of the disease can be inferred from what the 8 to 16 year olds tell about their disease in the interview and from what the 4 to 7 year olds tell about this in the hospital play. Table 7.9.1 presents the specific knowledge the children in the different age groups possess. It must be noted here that it concerns the spontaneous answers to ques-

Table 7.9.1
Percentage of children in different age groups possessing specific knowledge of the disease.

Knowledge of the disease	Age groups		
	Data from the hospital play	Data from the interview	
	4-7 years (n=26) %	8-12 years (n=32) %	13-16 years (n=24) %
Seriousness	88	84	88
Long period of illness	50	59	63
Tumor/Growth/Medical term	19	72	92
Malignant (cells)	0	3	21
Cancer	4	50	71
Possibility of metastasis	4	33	50
Possibility of relapse or recurrence	19	69	83
Possibility of not getting better	15	72	83
Possibility of dying	15	66	79

tions formulated in general terms such as: "What kind of illness do you (did you) have?" and "Is it bad (serious) or not so bad (serious)?"
Similar questions are asked in the hospital play concerning the sick child (doll). Detailed questions for determining the child's available and missing knowledge have not been asked. Such direct questions are ethically objectionable because in this way the child could actually receive information about his or her illness from the interviewer, which he or she did not previously possess. As can be seen in Table 7.9.1, there is a distinct increase in specific knowledge about the disease as the child is older. There is a strong relationship between the child's age and total knowledge about the disease ($r=.73$, $p<.01$). If we compare the data of the middle and oldest age group in Table 7.9.1 with the data in Table 7.1.2, there is a high degree of correspondence between the specific information about the disease which the parents have given and the specific knowledge about the disease which the children possess. For the youngest age group the correspondence is considerably lower. This probably has to be attributed to the different method of measurement used in this age group. These children had not been asked a direct question about what disease they have or had themselves, but knowledge about the disease has been inferred from the nature of the disease which they project onto the sick child (doll) in the hospital play and from further knowledge which emerges during the play. But among the entire group of children, there is still a fairly strong relationship between the amount of information about the disease which one or both parents have given to the child and the total knowledge about the disease which the child possesses ($r=.53$, $p<.01$). A few of the 8 to 12 year old children call the disease cancer in the hospital play, but do not use this term when they are describing their own illness in the interview. The concept in the literature called "middle knowledge" is applicable to the reactions of these children. For example, an eleven year old girl recounts in the interview:

> "I have a tumor on my eye. That's a little bump and if it stays there then you'll get it everywhere and then you'll die. Some of the other children in hospital have cancer. Luckily I don't. Sometimes those other children had the same as I did but on another spot...Yeah, we sometimes talked about this together. About diseases that we all have, cancer, and...yeah, it's a very bad disease, aye."

One moment the girl denies she has cancer but the next moment she hints she is aware of having the same disease as the other chil-

Table 7.9.2
Percentage of parents who think their child is aware of the seriousness of the disease.

The child's awareness of the seriousness	Mothers (n=81) %	Fathers (n=78) %
Yes	57	62
Don't know	6	10
No	37	28

dren. Most noticeable in Table 7.9.1 is the high percentage of children who call the disease bad or serious. This percentage is also high among the youngest children. The 8 to 16 year old children were asked what is bad or serious about the illness. Most of the children could indicate that the illness is bad or serious because you can die of it (see Table 7.9.1).

Table 7.9.2 presents the answers of parents to the question whether they think their child is aware of the seriousness of the disease. More than half of the mothers and almost two-thirds of the fathers think their child is aware of the seriousness of the disease. A few parents indicate they don't know whether their child is aware of the seriousness of the disease. There is a clear relationship with the child's age. As the child is older, the parents more often think the child is aware of the seriousness of the disease ($r=.38$, $p<.01$ for the mothers and $r=.54$, $p<.01$ for the fathers).

8. Exploration of the intensity of emotional reactions, situational factors, and intrapersonal factors

8.1. The intensity of the emotional reactions of the child and the parents

By intensity of emotional reactions, we refer to both the frequency with which certain feelings are experienced (e.g. how often is the child anxious?) and the strength of these feelings (e.g. is the child somewhat anxious or very anxious?). In this section we discuss the results concerning the intensity with which children with cancer and their parents experience unpleasant and pleasant emotions. The degree to which the parents assess the behavior of their child as anxious, depressive, rebellious, and introvert is also discussed here. The intensity of the children's behavioral problems, which are conceived to be expressions of emotional problems, is explained in this section as well. The most significant results can be summarized as follows:

- Children with cancer between 8 and 12 years old are more anxious, more depressed, and have a more negative self-esteem than healthy peers.
- Children with cancer between 4 and 7 years old are more anxious and more depressed than 8 to 12 year old children with cancer. The latter, in turn, are more anxious, more depressed, and have a more negative self-esteem than 13 to 16 year old children with cancer.
- Parents report that their child is not very anxious and not very depressed. This assessment by the parents shows little or no correspondence with the degree of anxiety and depression which the child itself reports.
- Parents more often assess their child's behavior as rebellious

than as anxious or depressed. However, this rebelliousness seems to be partly symptomatic of the child's anxiety and depression.
- The parents assess their child as being fairly open.
- Spontaneous expressions of fear of death by the children rarely occur.
- The intensity of positive and negative feelings which the 8 to 12 year old children with cancer experience towards their mother, father, and siblings does not differ from healthy peers nor from 13 to 16 year old children with cancer.
- According to the parents, more than three-quarters of the children display at least one behavioral problem to a greater or lesser extent. Almost three-quarters of the children have sleeping problems; almost one-fifth of the children have bed-wetting problems, but this behavior cannot be called deviant; more than half of the children have eating problems and this problem is more serious among them than among other sick children; one-third of the children have problems at school.
- Parents of children with cancer do not exhibit more psychological and psychosomatic stress reactions and anxiety than a randomly selected sample from the Dutch population.
- The use of sleeping pills and sedatives, as well as the frequency of the parents' visits to the family doctor for their own complaints, is not deviant.
- The mothers exhibit more psychological and psychosomatic stress reactions and go to the family doctor more often for their own complaints than the fathers.
- On the whole, the parents appear to be relatively optimistic about the chances of a cure for their child and are not frequently troubled by thoughts of losing their child.
- Both the mothers and fathers project feelings of anxiety, insecurity, and feelings of helplessness, but also positive feelings to quite a large extent, while feelings of loneliness and isolation, anxiety about not being able to keep it up, and feelings of guilt are projected less often.

The means and standard deviations of the scales used to measure the emotional reactions of children and parents are presented in Appendix V. The means and standard deviations of the different age groups of children are also included here, as well as the scale range of each scale. The latter is the minimum and maximum score which can be reached on the scale. Appendix VI presents the correlations between the behavioral assessment scales and the problem behavior assessment scales of the parents, on the one hand, and the anxiety and depression scales of the children, on the other hand. Differences in means between the children in different age groups and between the fathers and mothers have been tested for statistical significance using t-tests. On some of the scales, the scores of the children and parents can be compared with the scores of healthy peers or other adults. This has also been done with t-tests. Whenever possible, we have compared the intensity of the children's behavioral problems with data on healthy children or other sick children.

The results are described in detail below and, if relevant, illustrated by qualitative data from the interview.

How anxious are children with cancer?

Comparison with healthy peers. A comparison of the anxiety level of the children with cancer and the anxiety level of healthy peers is possible to a limited extent only. The STAIC Anxiety Trait scale and the STAIC Anxiety-State scale have not yet been studied on a representative sample of Dutch children. However, data are available on 55 Dutch boys aged 11 and 12 years (Bakker & Van Wieringen, 1985). The scores of the 8 to 12 year old children are the most eligible ones for comparing with the scores of this group of healthy peers. Because no sex differences were found in these questionnaires (see section 8.2), the scores of the girls in this age group are included in the comparison. The 8 to 12 year old children with cancer score significantly higher on the anxiety trait scale (t=5.28, p<.01). On the anxiety-state scale, the scores can be compared with the scores of healthy peers to whom the scale has been administered under neutral conditions and under stressful conditions. When comparing the means under neutral conditions, the 8 to 12 year old children with cancer score significantly higher (t=2.54, p<.05). There is no significant difference with the mean under stressful conditions. These findings show that children with cancer between 8 and 12 years old describe themselves as more anxious than healthy peers. They appear to be anxious more often (higher anxiety trait). Moreover, they respond with an equally high level of anxiety(-state) in the interview situation as healthy peers who are exposed to stressful conditions, and with a higher level of anxiety(-state) than healthy peers who are exposed to neutral conditions. Thus it can be inferred that the children have experienced the interview situation and talking about the disease as anxiety-arousing. A more precise indication of the intensity of the children's anxiety is not possible because, for example, data on percentile scores of a standardization sample are not available. The following data may give an impression. On the anxiety trait scale, the 8 to 12 year old children with cancer score an average of 7 points higher than the comparison group. The scale range is 20-60 and 28% of the children have a score of 45 or higher. On the anxiety-state scale, the 8 to 12 year old children with cancer score an average of 2 points higher than the comparison group under neutral conditions. This scale also has a range of 20-60. None of the children reach a score of more than 43 on this scale.

Differences in anxiety level by age group. The means and standard deviations for the different age groups are presented in Appendix V. If we compare the means of the 8 to 12 year olds with the 13 to 16 year olds, the younger group scores significantly higher on the anxiety trait scale (t=2.81, p<.01), but there is no difference in the means on the anxiety-state scale. It may be inferred that the adolescents with cancer (13 to 16 year olds) are less (often) anxious than the younger children (8 to 12 year olds), but they experience the interview situation as anxiety-arousing to a similar extent. When talking about the disease during the interview, they respond with the same degree of anxiety as the younger children. The degree of anxiety and tension has also been assessed by the latency and the number of blocks in the interview and hospital play. The latency (hesitations or silences before a question is answered) is the same in all age groups. In the hospital play, the number of blocks (no response or the answer "I don't know" as the only response) is significantly higher among the 4 to 7 year old children than among the 8 to 12 year old children (t=2.79, p<.01). There is no significant difference in the interview between the number of blocks among the 8 to 12 year olds and the number of blocks among the 13 to 16 year olds. In the hospital play, the 4 to 7 year old children project significantly more fear of pain and procedures (needles, infusions, operations, etc.) than the 8 to 12 year old children (t=2.37, p<.05). Fear of pain and procedures was not measured in the adolescents, but they also have these fears, as presented in section 8.2. In the hospital play, the 4 to 7 year old children also project significantly more feelings of diffuse anxiety than the 8 to 12 year old children (t=2.35, p<.05). The sick child (doll) is afraid but the younger children are less capable of indicating what frightens them, or they mention ghosts or scary sounds as the cause of anxiety.

Anxiety and frustration about the disease in the adolescents. An impression of the degree to which adolescents (13 to 16 year olds)

project feelings of disease-related anxiety and frustration, can be attained by comparing the mean score to the scale range (minimum to maximum score which can be reached on this scale; see Appendix V). It may be inferred that the frequency with which adolescents attribute these feelings to fellow-sufferers is not extreme. A few specific feelings of anxiety and frustration are projected to quite a large extent. It involves anxiety about hospital admissions and checkups, as well as frustration due to physical restrictions and changes in appearance. The percentage of adolescents who often or almost always consider these feelings to be present in other adolescents with cancer is as follows:
Anxiety about being admitted into hospital again (59%);
Nervous when you have to go to the hospital for a checkup (58%);
Feeling bad because you look different due to the treatment (54%);
Anger because you can't do certain things anymore (50%).

The children's fear of death. For ethical reasons we decided not to ask the children directly whether and how often they experience fear of death. Therefore we must rely on the child's spontaneous remarks about this. Despite the fact that quite a large number of children give evidence of being aware that they might die of the disease and that fellow patients have died of the disease (see section 7.9), spontaneous remarks about the children's fear of death rarely occur. Among the 4 to 12 year olds, projection of fear of death is explicitly stated by only a few children (9%). The children do answer the question in the hospital play about whether the child (doll) is sometimes afraid and why this is the case, by: "It's afraid that things aren't going so well for him/her" or "It's afraid that something terrible will happen to him/her". But there are only one or two children who go as far as this seven year old boy:

> "Well, he's scared because it's so bad what he's got, that he will never get better. That the doctor will not be able to make him better and, um, that something terrible will happen to him ... that he, um, then, um, will die."

In the interview with the 8 to 16 year old children, spontaneous remarks about fear of death also rarely occur. In answer to the question what children think to be the worst thing about their illness, only a few children mention the possible fatal outcome of the disease. There are only two children who say they sometimes dream about dying. A ten year old girl (who died a few months after the study) says:

> "I dreamt a few times that I died. Then I woke up and had to cry a lot. Then Mommy came and she said: You aren't going to die. You'll get better. But I have also dreamt I was with Santa Claus in the hospital and that dream came true."

An eleven year old boy expresses a fear of his own death and projects this fear onto the whole of humankind:

> "Sometimes when I lie in bed I worry. Well, actually quite a lot. Then I think about the illness and about dying and about some other things. Then I'm also afraid of disasters and that sort of thing. That the whole world will die or something like that."

A few questions in the depression questionnaire and the anxiety trait scale refer, implicitly or explicitly, to death and fear of death. For the following questions, the percentage of 8 to 16 year old children who answered these questions in the affirmative is reported in brackets. I thought for awhile that I didn't want to live anymore (30%); Nowadays I often think that maybe I won't get very old (16%); I think more often lately that I would rather be dead (18%); I'm often scared that something bad will happen to me or to someone in our family (45%); I'm worried that something will happen to my parents (73%). It is not known how often healthy children answer these questions in the affirmative, but it can be inferred that many children with cancer think about death. Almost three-quarters of the children report they worry that something might happen to their parents. This can be seen as a projection of their own anxieties, but probably also reflects the children's feeling of vulnerability. In a situation where the children heavily rely on their parents' protection, it is conceivable that fear of losing them will be stronger.

How anxious is the child, according to the parents? On the whole, the parents believe that their child is not very anxious. If we relate the mean on the behavioral assessment scale *not anxious versus anxious behavior of the child* in relation to the scale range (see Appendix V), we see that both mothers and fathers perceive relatively little anxiety in their child. This can also be inferred from the percentage of parents whose scores lie at the extreme poles of this behavioral dimension. The percentage of parents whose scores lie at the poles *rather anxious* or *very anxious* is low (7% of the mothers and 6% of the fathers), while the percentage of parents whose scores lie at the poles *hardly ever anxious* or *not anxious at all* is rather high (41% of the mothers and 47% of the fathers). In contrast to the measures of anxiety in the children themselves, the anxiety which the parents perceive in the child is not related to the child's age. Furthermore, there is hardly any relationship between the degree of anxiety the parent perceives in the child and the degree of anxiety the children report themselves or project (see Appendix VI). A reason for this lack of correspondence between children and parents may be that the assessment of anxiety by the parent is not related to the child's defensiveness, while most measures of the child's anxiety are negatively correlated with defensiveness to quite a high degree. The parents probably infer the child's anxiety from his/her behavior, without being influenced by the child's tendency to deny his/her fears. The lack of correspondence cannot be blamed on a projection of the parents' own anxieties. There are no significant correlations between the anxiety measures of the parent and the anxiety measures of the child. The fact that parents judge their child's anxiety as being relatively low, while the children themselves, as explained above, do appear to be quite anxious, leads to the assumption that either the child tries to protect the parents and/or the parents try to protect themselves. Perhaps the children try to hide their anxiety from the parents and are fairly successful in this and/or the parents protect themselves because they cannot or do not want to see their child as anxious. We will return to this in the next section.

How depressed are children with cancer?

Comparison with healthy peers. It is possible to compare the degree of depression in children in our study to the degree of depression in healthy peers. It concerns the depression questionnaire (DQC) and the subscales of this questionnaire. This questionnaire has test norms based on a representative sample of Dutch boys and girls between the ages of 9 and 12 years (De Wit, 1985). The scores of the 8 to 12 year olds are the most eligible ones for comparison with the scores of this standardization group of healthy peers. The 8 to 12 year old children with cancer have a significantly higher total score on the depression questionnaire (t=3.07, p<.01); the children score an average of 8 points higher and 22% of the children score in the highest decile (score >44). The children in our study also score significantly higher on the subscale *negative self-esteem* (t=3.18, p<.01). There is no difference with the standardization group on the subscales *negative evaluation of the social environment* and *negative expectations for the future*. Children with cancer between the ages of 8 and 12 years describe themselves as more depressed than healthy peers and also have a more negative self-esteem. However, they do not have a more negative attitude towards their social environment and, remarkably enough, their expectations for the future are not more gloomy.

Differences in degree of depression in the three age groups. The means and standard deviations for the depression scales by age group are presented in Appendix V. The 8 to 12 year old children score significantly higher on the depression questionnaire than the 13 to 16 year old children. The youngest group has a significantly higher total score (t=2.25, p<.05) and a significantly higher score on the subscale *negative self-esteem* (t=2.48, p<.05). The groups do not differ significantly on the subscale *negative evaluation of the social environment* and *negative expectations for the future*. The younger children (8 to 12 year olds) show more depression and also exhibit more negative self-esteem than the older children (13 to 16 year olds). For the projective measures of depression, the 4 to 7 year old children are more depressed than the 8 to 12 year olds. In the hospital play, the youngest children project significantly more feelings of loneliness and isolation (t=3.90, p<.01), more feelings of frustration (t=2.46, p<.05), and more feelings of grief (t=2.04, p<.05). The younger children more often associate the situation created by the disease with being alone and missing parents, siblings, and friends, with frustrations about having to remain in bed and not being able to play, and with grief caused by these events.

Feelings of loneliness and isolation and feelings of pessimism in the adolescents. If we compare the mean score of the adolescents (13 to 16 year olds) on the projective measures of depression with the scale range (see Appendix V), we see that adolescents project feelings of loneliness and isolation and feelings of pessimism to quite a small degree. For example, only 8% of the adolescents indicate that fellow-sufferers often feel they are left to their own resources, and 29% of the adolescents indicate that fellow-sufferers almost never worry about the future.

How depressed is the child, according to the parents? On the whole, the parents see their child as not very depressed. This becomes clear if we look at the mean score of the parents on the behavioral assessment scale *cheerful versus depressive behavior of the child* in relation to the scale range (see Appendix V). Both the mothers and fathers perceive relatively little depressive behavior in their child. More evidence comes from the percentage of parents whose scores lie at the extreme poles of these behavioral dimensions. Some be-

Table 8.1.1
Percentage of parents whose scores lie at the extreme poles of behavioral dimensions on the behavioral assessment scale "cheerful versus depressive behavior of the child" (BAP-ChD).

Rather or very	Mothers (n=81) %	Fathers (n=78) %
Pessimistic	5	3
Optimistic	74	81
Unhappy	1	5
Happy	77	65
Gloomy	0	0
Cheerful	77	73
Lonely	1	4
Not lonely	67	62
Sad	0	1
High-spirited	79	78

havioral dimensions of this assessment scale are presented in Table 8.1.1. Here we see that a very low percentage of parents judge their child as being rather or very pessimistic, unhappy, gloomy, lonely, and sad, while a high percentage of parents judge their child as being rather or very optimistic, happy, cheerful, not lonely, and high-spirited.

In contrast to the depression measured in the children themselves, the parents' assessment of their child's depression is not related to the child's age. There is a low correspondence between the degree of depression which the parent perceives in the child and the degree of depression which the children themselves report and project. There are only a few significant correlations and these are low (see Appendix VI). There are no indications that parents project their own feelings of pessimism onto the child. There are no significant correlations between the measures of the child's depression and the degree of the parents' pessimism about the outcome of the disease. In spite of a somewhat higher correspondence between the parents' assessment of their child's depression and the depressive reactions reported by the child, once more it is striking that the parents appear to view the emotional experience of their child much too positively. This image deviates from the children's own perceptions, at least for the younger children. As we already noticed above, especially the younger children quite often describe themselves as rather depressed and/or project feelings of depression. Just like the child's anxiety, this might indicate that the children are hiding their feelings of depression from the parents and/or that this is a reaction of self-protection by the parents, because they do not want to or are unable to see their child as gloomy and depressed. Here we must also report the finding that there is no higher degree of correspondence between the parents' evaluation of the child's anxiety and depression and the degree of anxiety and depression which the children themselves indicate, if the parents actively ask about the child's emotional experience of the illness and/or express their own worries and grief to the child. Both the parents and children could be the cause. In the interview, the parents frequently mention that their child says little about his/her emotional experience if they ask about this directly but, for example, they can see from their child's games that the child is occupied with the illness and the hospital experiences. For example, a father of a six year old boy relates:

> "Awhile ago he played veterinarian. There was a sick rabbit. It had to eat its pills otherwise it would die. But if I ask him directly: And you, how are you feeling?, he just walks away."

A number of older children state in the interview that they are reluctant to talk with their parents about their emotional experience. A fourteen year old boy says:

> "I don't talk a lot with my father and mother. I like to keep it all to myself. It's difficult anyway when it all comes up again. That could last for years yet. You have to try to get over it yourself. Usually I can manage. If I have big problems then I talk to my parents. But if I have a dream which makes me lie awake all night and I lie there worrying, then I don't talk about it. Sometimes I tell them I had a dream but I don't say what it was about. Or I only say that I dreamt that I was sick again. That's enough for them."

The boy answers 'no' to the question from the interviewer whether his parents sometimes asked exactly what he had dreamt about. This shows that not only the children are reluctant to discuss emotionally-charged topics, but the parents as well.

The intensity of positive and negative feelings of the child towards the family members

The Family Relations Test has not yet been administered to a representative sample of Dutch children. Some tentative test norms are available for 6 to 11 year old boys and girls (Baarda et al., 1983), based on a few German and Dutch studies. If we compare the scores of the 8 to 12 year old children with cancer to the scores of these healthy peers, then we can conclude that the means do not differ significantly. This finding means that the intensity of positive and negative feelings experienced by the 8 to 12 year old children with cancer towards their mother, father, and siblings does not differ from the feelings of healthy peers. A comparison with healthy peers is not possible for the oldest age group (13 to 16 year olds) and the youngest age group (4 to 7 year olds). We would like to remark, however, that the experience of family relations of the 13 to 16 year old children with cancer does not differ from the experiences of the 8 to 12 year olds. There is no significant difference between the means of these two age groups.

The intensity of the child's behavioral problems

The children's rebelliousness. The degree to which parents assess their child to be depressed and anxious has already been explained in the previous sections. There we concluded that, in general, parents assess their child as quite cheerful and not very anxious. Regarding the other types of emotional behavior and specific behavioral problems which can be conceived to be expressions of emotional problems, we note, in the first place, that parents see more rebelliousness in their child. This becomes apparent if we compare the parents' mean score on the behavioral assessment scale *calm versus rebellious behavior of the child* with the scale range (see Appendix V). The percentage of parents whose scores lie at the extreme poles of these behavioral dimensions points to the same conclusion. Several behavioral dimensions of this assessment scale are presented in Table 8.1.2. Here we see that approximately one-fifth of the parents assess their child's behavior as rather or very rebellious, excited, and impatient. Quite a high percentage of parents feel their child's behavior is rather or very attention-demanding.

It was previously mentioned that the parents' assessment of the child's anxiety hardly corresponds at all with the anxiety which the child reports and projects. Therefore it is surprising that the parents' assessment of the child's rebelliousness is more strongly related to the anxiety which the child reports. Furthermore, the

Table 8.1.2
Percentage of parents whose scores lie at the extreme poles of behavioral dimensions on the behavioral assessment scales "calm versus rebellious behavior of the child" (BAP-CR) and "open versus introvert behavior of the child" (BAP-OI).

Rather or very	Mothers (n=81) %	Fathers (n=78) %
BAP-CR		
Rebellious	15	21
Obedient	22	21
Excited	18	21
Calm	21	21
Impatient	20	26
Patient	28	21
Attention-demanding	43	46
Wait-and-see	5	4
BAP-OI		
Open	62	55
Close	12	14
Extravert	64	56
Introvert	10	10

mothers' assessment about the child's rebelliousness is more strongly related to the depression which the child reports. This is apparent from the level of the correlations in Appendix VI. This means that the rebelliousness and agitation which the parents perceive in their child are probably partly symptomatic of the child's anxiety and depression. The fact that parents more often interpret their child's behavior as rebellious rather than anxious and gloomy, reinforces the impression that the parents are protected by the child and/or that the parents protect themselves.

The child's introversion. On the behavioral assessment scale *open versus introvert behavior of the child*, the parents assess their child as fairly open. This can be seen if we compare the mean score on this scale with the scale range (see Appendix V). This is also shown in Table 8.1.2 which presents the percentage of parents whose scores lie at the extreme poles of these behavioral dimensions. The percentage of parents who assess their child as rather or very open and extravert is quite high, while the percentage of parents who assess their child as rather or very close and introvert is low. This implies that parents assume they are well informed about what their child is occupied with due to the child's openness. The too positive view held by the parents of the child's anxiety and depression, and the fact that parents assess their child's behavior as rebellious while this is probably partly symptomatic of the child's anxiety and depression, raises doubt about the accuracy of this assumption by the parents.

The children's sleeping problems. In the case of almost three-quarters of the children (71%), one or both parents report the occurrence of sleeping problems. These problems consist of difficulties in going to sleep and/or often waking up and/or having bad dreams. Sleeping problems do not appear to be related to the child's anxiety or depression. The degree of the child's sleeping problems which the parents report does not correlate significantly with the anxiety or depression which the child reports or projects (see Appendix VI).

Bed-wetting by the children. According to one or both parents, 18% of the children have bed-wetting problems at least once a month, and 15% of the children more frequently. Bed-wetting is mainly a problem among the younger children, but one-third of the children with bed-wetting problems in our study is older than 7 years. Epidemiological research by De Jonge (1969) and Doleys (1977) gives an indication of the frequency with which this problem occurs among healthy children. De Jonge found that bed-wetting frequently (5-7 times a week) occurs in more than 1% of a population of Dutch children between the ages of 10 and 12. From American research by Doleys, it appeared that approximately 15% of the five year old children still regularly wet their bed, while this percentage gradually decreases to about 2% among the 12 to 14 year olds. If we compare the bed-wetting by children with cancer with these data we may assume that this problem does not occur more frequently in our group. However, there is a clear relationship between bed-wetting and the child's anxiety and depression. There are a number of significant positive correlations between the frequency of bed-wetting and the child's anxiety and depression variables (see Appendix VI).

The children's eating problems. One or both parents report eating problems for 59% of the children. These problems consist of eating too little and/or being too choosy and/or having a negative attitude when eating. For a few children eating problems concern excessive eating during the periods when they use corticosteroids. Messer (1979) quotes research which demonstrates that, in a general pediatric practice, approximately 25% of the children have eating problems. This percentage is considerably higher in our study and has remarkably little association with specific disease variables, as will be discussed in section 8.2. Only the fathers report significantly more eating problems for children who are undergoing treatment, however, the correlation is low (see Appendix VII). There is no significant correlation between eating problems reported by the mother and the fact that the child is still undergoing treatment. From the mother's assessment, we see that eating problems occur just as often among children still receiving chemotherapy as among children whose treatment has been completed - sometimes a long time ago. In the interview, some children report that certain types of food and smells are permanently aversive to them because these are associated with the smell of medicine or the sickness and vomiting during treatments.

The children's problems at school. Regarding the child's problems at school, we did not examine the child's school achievements, but the frequency of school absenteeism which had not been caused by the child's physical condition, and the child's motivation for and pleasure in going to school. In the case of 30% of the children, one or both parents report that the child is not very motivated to go to school and/or dreads going to school and/or skips school even if the child does not feel ill or cannot go to school for other reasons. The frequency with which these problems arise is related to the child's specific disease characteristics (see Appendix VII), but almost not to the child's emotional reactions (see Appendix VI). The relationship between behavioral problems and the child's age will be discussed in section 8.2.

The intensity of the parents' emotional reactions

Psychological and psychosomatic stress reactions. The parents' scores on the Well-being scale *psychological stress reactions* and *psychosomatic stress reactions* can be compared with test norms established on the basis of a study among 1622 randomly chosen Dutch men and women between the ages of 16 and 60 years (Ormel, 1980a, 1980b). Because separate data for men and women are not available, the mean scores of the total group of parents (mothers plus fathers) were compared with the mean scores of the standardization group. The mean scores of the parents on the psychological stress reactions scale and on the psychosomatic stress reactions scale are not significantly different from the means of the standardization group. We can conclude that parents of children with cancer do not report more psychological and psychosomatic stress reactions than persons representing an average of the Dutch population. But the mothers do report significantly more psychological stress reactions than the fathers (t=4.48, p<.01) and also significantly more psychosomatic stress reactions (t=3.82, p<.01). This corresponds with Ormel's (1980a) findings. He also found that women report significantly more unpleasant feelings and physical complaints than men.

Anxiety during the interview. The mean scores of the mothers and fathers on the anxiety-state scale (SRQ-AS) can be compared with the mean and decile scores of a group of almost 400 randomly selected men and women from Leiden between the ages of 16 and 70 years, who completed the questionnaire under neutral conditions (Van der Ploeg, 1981). The mean scores on the anxiety-state scale of the mothers and fathers are not significantly different from the means of the women or men in the comparison group. There are no significant differences either if we compare the scores in the highest deciles. Thus we can conclude that being interviewed did not constitute an anxiety-arousing situation for the parents. But the mothers score significantly higher on the anxiety-state scale than the fathers (t=2.98, p<.01). This corresponds with the results of Van der Ploeg et al. (1980) who also found that women score higher than men on the anxiety-state scale.

The use of sleeping pills and sedatives. In the week prior to the study, 14% of the mothers and 6% of the fathers used sleeping pills and/or sedatives. This difference between the mothers and fathers is not significant. We can compare the use of pills by the parents, up to a point, with the data on medical consumption which Ormel (1980a) obtained from 181 persons (random sample of Dutch men and women between the ages of 21 and 65 years). This part of the study was conducted in 1977. In the month prior to the study, 11% of the respondents used sleeping pills and/or sedatives daily. We did not ask the parents whether they took these pills everyday, but the consumption of sleeping pills and/or sedatives in our group does not seem to deviate from the comsumption in the relatively small but representative sample of the Dutch population studied by Ormel.

The frequency of visits to the family doctor. Ormel (1980a) also obtained data from the above-mentioned group on the frequency of visits to the family doctor. On average, the family doctor was consulted three times a year. More than one-quarter (27%) had not visited the doctor in the past year and 10% went more than seven times a year. More data on the frequency of visits to the family doctor are available from the *Living conditions study* conducted by the CBS in 1980 among more than 2800 Dutch men and women of 18 years and older. The respondents were asked the question: "How often have you been to the family doctor during the past three months for your own complaints?". In the age category corresponding with those of the parents (25-54 years), 45% of the women and 35% of the men had consulted the family doctor at least once; 23% of the women and 18% of the men had gone once; 6% of the women and 5% of the men more than three times. In our study, 46% of the mothers and 29% of the fathers had been to the family doctor during the three months prior to the study; 22% of the mothers and 22% of the fathers had been once; 5% of the mothers had gone more than three times. The fathers consulted the family doctor a maximum of two times. The frequency of visits is significantly higher for mothers than for fathers ($t=3.00$, $p<.01$). The frequency of consulting the doctor by the mothers and fathers does not deviate from the frequency of visits to the doctor in the Dutch population. In this context, it may be mentioned that two parents in our study (one mother and one father) were declared unfit to work and five fathers (6%) did not go to work at the time of the study due to illness. For two fathers this had been the case for more than half a year. These numbers are not very different from the national average either.

Pessimism about the course of the child's illness. No direct comparison with other groups is possible on the scale *pessimism about the course of the child's illness*. The scale refers to feelings of pessimism in the current stage of the child's disease. As can be inferred from the means in Appendix V, the parents turn out to be reasonably optimistic about their child's chances of being cured and are not frequently occupied with thoughts about losing their child. There is no signficiant difference between mothers and fathers regarding pessimism about the course of the child's illness in the current stage of the disease.

Table 8.1.3 presents the distribution of the item scores on three pessimism scales referring to the parents' pessimism in different stages of the child's disease. Because the scores for the group of mothers are very similar to those of the group of fathers, the percentages of the entire group of parents are shown. In the Table we

Table 8.1.3
Distribution of scores on the pessimism scales for the parents (n=159).

	Pessimism about the course of the child's illness		
	When learning the diagnosis	At the beginning of treatment	In the current stage of the disease
	%	%	%
Pessimistic	69	27	9
Neither pessimistic nor optimistic	10	7	16
Optimistic	21	66	75
Thoughts about losing the child	88	77	78
Thoughts about losing the child everyday	67	53	21

see a distinct shift from predominant pessimism when learning the child's diagnosis, to predominant optimism when the child's treatment starts. In the current stage of the disease (at the time of the study), optimism about a favorable outcome of the disease is even stronger. Many parents think about the possibility of losing the child, but these thoughts become less persistent as time passes. This thought is still in the minds of one-fifth of the parents everyday in the current stage of the disease. The questions about optimism or pessimism and about thoughts of losing the child in the initial stage of the disease are retrospective, i.e. they are about the memory which the parents have of this period. It is remarkable that one-third of the parents report they were not occupied everyday with thoughts of losing their child in the period between learning the diagnosis and the start of the child's treatment. This period covers an average of seven days in our study. This indicates a much described reaction of denial and numbness caused by the shock of this announcement. In the interview a father says:

> "I didn't realize I might lose him. I knew it was serious but it hadn't really dawned on me. I hadn't felt it deep down inside me yet."

The shift from predominant pessimism when the diagnosis is announced to predominant optimism when the treatment starts, seems to be a reflection of an attitude of optimism or pessimism which the parents perceive in the doctor. When asked the question whether the referring pediatrician was optimistic or pessimistic about the chances of a cure for the child at the moment this person told them the diagnosis, one-third of the parents (33%) responded that they felt the doctor was pessimistic. Almost one-quarter of the parents (24%) felt that the doctor was neither pessimistic nor optimistic, and 43% felt that the doctor was optimistic about the chances of curing the child. During the encounter with the pediatrician in the Children's Oncology Center, when the diagnosis was definitely confirmed and the treatment plan was discussed with the parents, only 9% of the parents felt the doctor was pessimistic about the chances of curing the child, 19% felt the doctor was neither pessimistic nor optimistic, and almost three-quarters of the parents (72%) felt the doctor was optimistic. We can assume that the perception of optimism or pessimism in the doctor is biased by personal feelings of optimism or pessimism. Some parents are aware of this. One father says:

> "I actually had the feeling that the doctor in the Emma Kinder Ziekenhuis was rather pessimistic. But I think that depends on yourself too. If you're very pessimistic yourself, then you notice that more quickly in someone else. I was completely shattered. The first few weeks I was a wreck. In my mind I had already delivered the funeral speech. I had a friend once with childhood cancer and I saw the agony he had to go through."

The offer of treatment opportunities which puts the possibility of control of the disease in a new perspective, turns out to be an important factor when estimating the doctor's optimism or pessimism. Referral to another hospital in itself seems to imply that the doctor cannot offer anything. Some referring doctors clearly show their pessimism, according to the parents. One father quotes the words of a referring pediatrician:

> "He said: She has to go to Amsterdam right away, or would you rather go home and take some pictures of her first?"

The pediatrician's optimistic attitude is not so much inferred by the parents from the promising predictions about the chances of curing the child, but rather from the fact that chances of a cure are not considered impossible. For example, one mother says:

> "In the Emma Kinder Ziekenhuis the doctor didn't want to say much about the chances. He said: it's fifty-fifty. We are doing our best and our goal is a cure. That gave us hope and confidence again. It gave us something to hold on to. Later you realize that a 50% chance of a cure is not really all that high."

Projection of situation-specific negative and positive feelings. We can find an indication of the degree to which the parents project negative and positive feelings specifically associated with the situation of parents of children with cancer if we look at the mean score of the parents in relation to the scale range (see Appendix V). This shows that parents score relatively high on the *anxiety and insecurity* scale and on the *helplessness* scale. The parents also score relatively high on the *positive feelings* scale. There is no significant difference on any of the scales between the mean score of the mothers and fathers. We can infer from this that both the mothers and fathers project feelings of anxiety and insecurity, feelings of helplessness, and also positive feelings to a rather high degree, while feelings of loneliness and isolation, anxiety about not being able to keep it up, and feelings of guilt are projected to a lesser degree. Table 8.1.4 shows the percentage of parents who hold the opinion that fellow-sufferers (other parents of children with cancer) harbor feelings specifically related to the situation created by the disease, quite often or seldom. Because the percentages are almost identical for the mothers and fathers, they are reported for the entire group of parents.

As the Table shows, 30% of the parents hold the opinion that feelings of anger about the lack of understanding from the social environment are frequently experienced by other parents of children with cancer. As the disease has been diagnosed longer ago, the treatment has been finished, and the disease symptoms are no longer obvious from the child's physical appearance, particularly the mothers project these feelings to a high degree (see section 8.2). In the interview, a number of them spontaneously report their own experiences about the lack of understanding and sympathy from those around them. A mother of an eight year old girl relates:

> "As long as she was very thin and bald, they could understand your worries. But now they say: Come on, she looks fine."

Table 8.1.4
Percentage of parents who score in the categories often/almost always or sometimes/almost never (n=159) on items representing situation-specific feelings (IBP).

	Other parents experience this	
Items on the scales	often/almost always %	sometimes/almost never %
Loneliness and isolation:		
Anger about the lack of understanding from those around you	30	70
The feeling that you don't belong anymore	4	96
The feeling that you've been shut out everywhere	6	94
Anxiety and insecurity:		
Insecurity about the outcome of the disease	85	15
Grief at the thought of losing your child	72	28
Anxiety that you will lose your child	69	31
Positive feelings:		
The feeling that you are more aware of life	84	16
The feeling that you can immensely enjoy the little things	67	33
The feeling that you can see the relativity of things much better	60	40
Happiness when you see your child enjoying him or herself	95	5
The feeling that the family has grown closer together	73	27
Feelings of helplessness:		
Feeling helpless because you can't do anything about the situation	85	15
Grief that your child has to undergo such terrible treatment	88	12
Grief that your child has to suffer	89	11
Having to watch while your child is in pain	88	12
Anger that your child had to have this fate	41	59
Anxiety about not being able to keep it up:		
The feeling that you are going to break down	18	82
Anxiety about not being able to keep it up	23	77
Feelings of guilt:		
The feeling that you have done things or have omitted things which might have influenced the development of your child's disease	21	79
Wondering whether you were too late in noticing that there was something seriously wrong with your child	35	65

A mother of a five year old girl relates:

> "She went through a period when everytime she came home from the hospital she would scream with fright at night. One time the neighbours came to our door and asked: Are you battering your child, or what?"

Sometimes the parents indicate that understanding and sympathy from others depends on their own attitude. For example, one mother says:

> "The family doctor had advised us to tell as few people as possible about what was going on. So we only said: there's something wrong with her blood. But after awhile people started to suspect things. Then I had an inner struggle. You had to start telling lies to people. I also had a fight with my husband because he felt we had to get our stories right. Then I decided I'd better tell the truth anyhow. Then you get a lot more understanding from other people because they had not dared to ask anything anymore."

Although feelings of uncertainty about the outcome of the disease and feelings of anxiety and grief at the thought of losing the child are projected by the parents to a fairly high degree (see Table 8.1.4), we did not observe any signs of an advanced process of anticipatory grief in the parents in our study. The composition of the group could be a factor because dying children did not participate in our study. Some of the children had a very poor prognosis but had not yet reached the stage at which curative treatment was terminated. Some parents indicate that, at the beginning, they started to emotionally withdraw from the child. This is especially the case if the child has practically been given a death sentence. A mother relates:

> "Here in the (regional) hospital the doctor initially said it was benign. Then he said we had to prepare for the worst, that it was malignant and there was nothing more to be done about it. He asked whether we had other children. Thank goodness, he said. The first few weeks it seemed as if the child wasn't mine. I was present at all the tests but it was as if I was an outsider. It was just like walking around in a dream. Then we went to the Emma Kinder Ziekenhuis. There they told us he had a chance and they thought they could do

something about it. It wasn't until weeks later that I thought: After all, he is my child. I have to go on."

The offer of treatment and the perspective of a chance of a cure for the child must have been of paramount importance in halting this process of emotional withdrawal. Anticipatory grief reactions in the form of defiance, grief, and a gradual acceptance of the possibility that one may lose the child can be observed in many parents. A father of a five year old boy (his only child) describes these reactions as follows:

> "It was a terrible blow for me when I heard what was wrong with him. It was like someone threw a stone through a window which cannot be repaired anymore. It made me cry. It's so unfair to the boy. Later on I managed to leave it all to science and to Our Heavenly Father."

8.2. The influence of biographical and disease characteristics on the communication style and the emotional reactions

The influence of biographical and disease characteristics on the parents' communication style and on the emotional reactions of the parents and children have been tested by performing Pearson correlations and univariate variance analyses. Although correlations do not indicate a causal relationship, we use the terms influence and effect of the biographical and disease characteristics on the communication style and on the emotional reactions. We consider it impossible that there could be an influence or effect in the opposite direction, i.e. that communication style and emotional reactions could have an influence or effect on biographical and disease characteristics. The main results are summarized as follows.

Biographical characteristics and the communication style. Biographical characteristics such as sex and birth rank of the child, or sex, age, education, and socio-economic status of the parent hardly have any influence on the parents' communication style. The child's age, on the other hand, has a very clear effect. Older children are given more information about the disease by their parents at an early stage, but younger children turn to their parents more often to talk about the disease, and the parents themselves talk to the child more often if the child is young.

Disease characteristics and communication style. The specific disease characteristics of the child hardly appear to have any influence on the parents' communication style. The nature of the diagnosis (tumor or leukemia), the nature of the prognosis (good or poor), having or having had a relapse or recurrence (return of disease symptoms), the success of treatment (being in initial remission or in subsequent remission), duration of the treatment, the number of hospital admissions, and the number of days in hospital all have no effect on the parents' communication style. The way information is given about the disease, the communication about the emotional experience, and the communication about the disease during the current stage of the disease are not related to these disease characteristics of the child. The latter aspect of communicaton is the only one which is influenced by the time since diagnosis, whether or not the child is still undergoing treatment, the frequency of visits to the clinic, and the physical-visible impairments as a consequence of the disease and/or treatment. Children take the initiative to talk about the disease with their parents more often if cancer has been diagnosed relatively recently, if they are still undergoing treatment, if they have to go to the clinic often for treatment and/or checkups, and if the consequences of the disease and/or treatment include physical restrictions and are visible in the child's appearance. Under these conditions the parents also take the initiative to talk with their child about the disease more often.

Biographical characteristics and emotional reactions. The effect of biographical characteristics on the child's emotional reactions are almost exclusively limited to the child's age. The younger the child, the greater the anxiety, depression, and behavioral problems. For the parents, the parent's sex is the most important factor. Compared with the fathers, the mothers show more psychological and psychosomatic stress reactions and more anxiety during the interview, and they consult the family doctor more often for their own complaints.

Disease characteristics and emotional reactions. The specific disease characteristics of the child appear to have remarkably little influence on the emotional reactions of both the children and parents. The entire situational context, determined by the child's cancer, seems to have a greater influence than differences which emerge from the specific disease and treatment conditions of the child.
Most of the child's anxiety and depression variables either turn out not to be related at all to disease characteristics or only related to a

single disease characteristic. The same applies to the child's behavioral problems and to how the child experiences family relations. Where disease characteristics do play a role, their influence is most evident on fear of pain and procedures, feelings of loneliness and isolation, and the child's problems at school. An influence of disease characteristics on the child's self-esteem and feelings towards the mother and siblings can also be observed.

Fear of pain and procedures is stronger among the 4 to 12 year old children if the child is still undergoing treatment and has to go to the clinic often for treatment and/or checkups. This fear is also stronger in children with leukemia. In addition to the frequency of the child undergoing painful procedures (e.g. children with leukemia regularly have bone marrow aspirations and lumbar punctures), the effectiveness of treatment also seems to play a role. Fear of pain and procedures happens to be stronger in children who have or have had a relapse or recurrence, but is less prevalent in children who are in their first continuous remission. These findings cannot be attributed to treatment duration. For children who have had a relapse or recurrence, treatment duration almost always increases, but this factor does not play a role regarding fear of pain and procedures. The same disease characteristics which influence the fear of pain and procedures appear to have an identical influence on the feelings of loneliness and isolation (among the 4 to 12 year olds) and on the child's problems at school (for all age groups). Treatment duration does play a role here. Feelings of loneliness and isolation and problems at school become stronger as the child's treatment duration increases. The problems at school involve diminished motivation for and lessened pleasure in going to school and involve school absenteeism not caused by physical conditions. The time since diagnosis and the duration of the treatment have a negative effect on the self-esteem of the 8 to 16 year old children. The children's self-esteem is more negative as the child has been diagnosed longer ago and the treatment is going on or has been going on for a longer period.

Regarding the experience of family relations, the disease characteristics mainly affect the 4 to 7 year old's negative and positive feelings towards siblings. Among the 8 to 16 year olds, they mainly influence negative feelings towards the mother. The younger children experience more positive and less negative feelings towards their siblings if their prognosis is poor and they have to go to the hospital often for treatment and/or checkups. They also experience less negative feelings towards their siblings if the disease and/or treatment cause physical restrictions and visible disfigurements, but these feelings increase as the child has been diagnosed longer ago and the treatment takes or has taken longer. The older children experience more negative feelings towards the mother if their prognosis is poor and they undergo or have undergone long-lasting clinical treatment and many hospital admissions.

Although the above findings create the impression that specific disease and treatment conditions considerably influence the child's emotional reactions, it should be remarked that most of the anxiety and depression variables and most of the child's behavioral problems are not influenced at all or are only influenced by a single disease characteristic. A more detailed presentation of the results in the next sections will explain this.

Just as in the case of the children, the influence of disease characteristics on the parents' emotional reactions appears to be quite small. Moreover, the findings among the mothers differ considerably from those among the fathers. For example, the mothers' feelings of pessimism are stronger if the child has leukemia, if the child has or has had a relapse or recurrence, and if the child is or has been treated for a long time. As is the case for the mothers, the fathers' feelings of pessimism increase if the child has or has had a relapse or recurrence. But these feelings are also stronger in the fathers if the child still has to go to hospital for treatment and/or checkups frequently and they decrease if the child is in initial remission or is in remission again after a relapse or recurrence. Prolonged clinical treatment is associated only among the mothers with increased psychological and psychosomatic stress reactions. Among the fathers, psychosomatic stress reactions are only related to the time since the child's diagnosis. As the child has been diagnosed longer ago, these reactions by the fathers increase. Furthermore, only the mothers' feelings of loneliness and isolation are influenced by the disease characteristics of the child. These feelings are less evident if the child is still undergoing treatment and if the disease and/or treatment cause physical restrictions and visible disfigurements. However, the mothers' feelings of loneliness and isolation increase as the child has been diagnosed longer ago. The other emotion variables of the parents do not appear to be related to disease characteristics at all or only to a few.

On the whole, most of the significant relationships described above are not very strong, not for the children and certainly not for the parents. The results are comprehensively presented below, by biographical variable and by disease variable. First, we will describe the effect of these variables on the parents' communication style, then on the children's emotion variables, and lastly, on the parents' emotional variables.

The influence of biographical and disease characteristics on the parents' communicaton style

The biographical and disease characteristics of the child have been related to the communication style of one or both parents as well as to the communication style of the group of mothers and the group of fathers separately. The biographical variables of the parents have only been related to the communication style of that parent.

Sex, age, and birth rank of the child. The child's sex is slightly related to one aspect of the communication style, this being the expression of worry to the child by one or both parents ($r=.26$, $p<.05$). The parents express their worries more often to girls than to boys. This relationship is not significant for the group of mothers and the group of fathers separately. The child's age has a stronger relationship with the parents' communication style. Table 8.2.1 presents the correlations between the child's age and the communication style, which are significant either for the communication style of one or both parents or for the group of mothers or the group of fathers separately. As the child is older, one or both parents have given more information about the diagnosis and prognosis to the child in the initial stage of the disease. If the point in time at which parents have given information about the diagnosis and prognosis is not taken into consideration, then the correlations between age and giving information are about the same. This means that older children have received more information about their disease from the parents anyway than younger children. The relationship between age and being informed about the diagnosis also applies to the group of mothers and the group of fathers separately. With respect to information about the prognosis, it only applies to the group of fathers and not to the group of mothers.

Thus older children have already received more information from their parents in the initial stage of their disease, but in the current stage of the disease they take the initiative less frequently to talk with their parents about the disease. As the child is younger, it turns more to the parents (both to the mother and to the father) to talk about the illness. The parents themselves also take the initiative to talk about the illness more often if the child is young. By the way, this only applies if the communication style of one or both parents is taken into consideration. This does not apply to the group of mothers and group of fathers separately. With respect to the remaining communication variables, the correlations with the child's age are weak and not significant. Thus the child's age does

Table 8.2.1
Pearson correlations (r) between the child's age and the communication variables (CSP) of one or both parents (n=82), of the mothers (n=81), and of the fathers (n=78).

	The child's age		
	Communication style		
	of one or both parents	of the mothers	of the fathers
Communication variables	r	r	r
Information about the diagnosis	.43**	.36**	.23*
Information about the prognosis	.39**	.21	.32**
Communication about the disease at the child's initiative	-.44**	-.32**	-.34**
Communication about the disease at the parent's initiative	-.25*	-.12	-.19

* = p<.05
** = p<.01

not influence the parental communication about the child's emotional experience, about the expression of worry and grief to the child, or the parents' habit of talking freely about the disease in the presence of the child. The effect of the child's birth rank has been tested by performing a univariate variance analysis. There does not appear to be a birth rank effect on the parents' communication style, neither on the communication style of one or both parents nor on the communication style of the group of mothers and group of fathers separately.

Sex and age of the parent. There is only one aspect of the communication style that has a significant relationship with the sex of the parent and this is the expression of grief (r=.35, p<.01). Mothers express grief to their child more often than fathers. The parent's age also has only one significant relationship with the parent's communication style. Children take the initiative to talk about the disease with a parent more often as the parent is younger (r=-.33, p<.01). This negative correlation is not surprising as this finding also applied to the children (younger children take the initiative more often to talk with parents about the disease than older children) and there is a fairly strong relationship between the child's age and the parent's age (r=.61, p<.01). It is more remarkable that the parents' age does not correlate either with information about the diagnosis and prognosis, or with communication about the disease at the parent's initiative. These communication variables did correlate significantly with the child's age. The correlations for the parents are in the same direction but they are weak and not significant.

Education and socio-economic status of the parent. There does not appear to be any relationship at all between the education or socio-economic status of the parent and the communication style. This means that the way the child is informed about the disease, the communication about the emotional experience, and the communication about the disease in the current stage of the disease are in no way influenced by the education or socio-economic status of the parent.

The disease characteristics of the child. There is only a very slight influence of the specific disease characteristics of the child on the parents' communication style. Disease characteristics such as nature of the diagnosis (tumor or leukemia), nature of the prognosis (good or poor), having or having had a relapse or recurrence, being in continuous first remission or in subsequent remission, treatment duration, the number of hospital admissions, and the number of days in hospital do not appear to have any effect on the communication style of one or both parents or on the communication style of the group of mothers and the group of fathers separately. A number of disease characteristics, i.e. time since diagnosis, undergoing treatment, frequency of clinic visits, and the physical-visible consequences of the disease and/or treatment only have a significant relationship with communication about the disease in the current stage of the disease. These correlations are presented in Table 8.2.2.

The correlations are not high so the relationship is weak. Nevertheless, the significant correlations mean that children take the initiative to talk about the disease with one or both parents and with the fathers more often as the time since diagnosis has been shorter, if the child is still undergoing treatment and still often has to go to the clinic for treatment and/or checkups, and if the disease and/or treatment cause physical restrictions and visible disfigurements (e.g. baldness). With the exception of the variable *still undergoing treatment*, these disease characteristics also influence the frequency with which one or both parents and the frequency with which the fathers take the initiative to talk with the child about the disease. Thus, under these conditions, communication between child and father increases. The communication between child and mother is not influenced by specific disease and treatment conditions.

Table 8.2.2
Pearson correlations (r) between several disease characteristics of the child and communication variables (CSP) of one or both parents (n=82), of the mothers (n=81), and of the fathers (n=78).

	Communication about the disease at the child's initiative			Communication about the disease at the initiative of		
	with one or both parents	with the mother	with the father	one or both parents	the mother	the father
Disease characteristics of the child	r	r	r	r	r	r
Time since diagnosis	-.27*	-.06	-.32**	-.27*	-.13	-.30**
Undergoing treatment	.31**	.18	.25*	.22	.09	.20
Frequency of visits to the clinic	-.34**	.22	.29*	.28*	.17	.31**
Physical-visible consequences of disease and/or treatment	.29**	.18	.25*	.30**	.19	.28*

* = p<.05
** = p<.01

The influence of biographical and disease characteristics on the child's emotional reactions

Biographical characteristics

The child's sex. With one exception, there is no effect of the child's sex on the emotional reactions of the children. Only fear of pain and procedures correlates significantly with the child's sex (r=.28, p<.05). Girls project more fear of pain and procedures than boys. There are no significant differences between boys and girls on all the other anxiety and depression variables. The experience of family relations and behavioral problems are not influenced by the child's sex either. To the extent that psychometric data on sex differences are available for our instruments, our findings correspond reasonably well with these data. With regard to the anxiety questionnaires (STAIC A-trait and STAIC A-state), Spielberger et al. (1973) found that girls score somewhat higher than boys, but not significantly higher. We found the same in our group. De Wit (1985) found that girls scored significantly higher than boys on the depression questionnaire (DQC), however, the difference appeared to be slight. In our study, girls also score somewhat higher than boys on the depression questionnaire but the difference is not significant. Finally, no clear sex differences emerge from the provisional standardization data of the Family Relations Test (Baarda et al., 1983). This appeared to be the same in our study.

The child's age. As already stated in section 8.1 the factor age clearly influences the children's emotional reactions. Table 8.2.3 and 8.2.4 present the significant correlations between age and anxiety and depression variables, and behavioral problems. A clear

Table 8.2.3
Pearson correlations (r) between the children's age and emotion variables.

Emotion variables of the child	n	Age of the child r
Anxiety variables:		
Anxiety trait (ST-AT) 8 to 16 year olds	56	-.33*
Blocks (ITW) 8 to 16 year olds	56	-.27*
Diffuse anxiety (HP-DA) 4 to 12 year olds	58	-.26*
Blocks (HP) 4 to 12 year olds	58	-.41**
Depression variables:		
Depression (DQC) 8 to 16 year olds	56	-.27*
Negative self-esteem (NE-se) 8 to 16 year olds	56	-.30*
Loneliness and isolation (HP-LI) 4 to 12 year olds	58	-.40**
Frustration (HP-F) 4 to 12 year olds	58	-.33*
Grief (HP-G) 4 to 12 year olds	58	-.29*

* = $p<.05$
** = $p<.01$

negative relationship can be seen between the child's age and the degree of the child's anxiety and depression. This is the case for both the 4 to 12 year old group and the 8 to 16 year old group.

As the child is younger, the 4 to 12 year olds project more diffuse anxiety, more feelings of loneliness and isolation, and more feelings of frustration and grief. The younger children become blocked more often during the hospital play. We see the same effect occurring in the 8 to 16 year olds. As the children are younger, they describe themselves as more anxious and more depressed, they have a more negative self-esteem, and they become blocked more often during the interview. Finally, the parents report more behavioral problems for children in the entire group as the child is younger. Both mothers and fathers mention more rebelliousness, bed-wetting, and problems at school for the younger children; the fathers report more eating problems for the younger children as well. The other anxiety and depression measures of the child, as well as anxiety and depression as assessed by the parents, correlate negatively with the child's age too, but these correlations are not significant. How the child experiences family relations and the child's positive feelings do not show any relationship with age.

Fear of pain and procedures has only been measured in the 4 to 12 year old children. No clear age effect emerges in this group. In the interview with the older children (8-16 year olds), adolescents appeared to have this fear just as much. A fourteen year old girl gives an example of this:

Table 8.2.4
Pearson correlations (r) between the child's age and behavioral problems of the children in all age groups, assessed by the mothers (n=81) and fathers (n=78).

	Age of the child	
	Behavioral problems of the child	
Behavioral problems of the child	assessed by the mother r	assessed by the father r
Calm versus rebellious behavior (BAP-CR)	-.32**	-.27*
Bed-wetting (PBAP-B)	-.39**	-.38**
Eating problems (PBAP-E)	-.18	-.31**
Problems at school (PBAP-SC)	-.26*	-.26*

* = $p<.05$
** = $p<.01$

"I never used to be scared of a needle. But finally I only had to see the needle to start screaming. The same with an infusion. It drove me really crazy just to see one in hospital. That's why I didn't want to have my last treatment. I didn't want anything anymore, didn't want to eat, drink, nothing. Then the doctor tried to convince me for an hour but I thought: you talk all you want to but I won't do it anymore. I sometimes dream about it now. About the hospital and infusions and then I wake up and start vomiting just like that."

There are hardly any psychometric data available on age effects for the instruments we used. On the depression questionnaire (DQC), De Wit (1985) did observe an age effect in spite of the limited age range of his standardization group (9-12 year olds). Younger children scored higher on the depression questionnaire than older children.

As the above discussion shows, the child's age does influence both a number of communication variables and quite a large number of emotion variables. For example, younger children receive less information about their disease from the parents and younger children are also more anxious, more depressed, and exhibit more behavioral problems. Thus the negative relationship between giving information, on the one hand, and anxiety, depression, and behavioral problems of the child, on the other hand (see section 6.1), may be based on a false relationship. That is, this may be caused by an age effect. After all, older children receive more information about their disease and older children also appear to be less anxious and less depressed, and appear to exhibit less behavioral problems. This age effect has been removed by performing partial correlations and, as reported in section 6.1, the negative relationship continues to exist between information, on the one hand, and anxiety, depression, and behavioral problems, on the other hand (the partial correlations are almost equal to the correlations). As children have received more information about their disease at an early stage, they are less anxious, less depressed, have a less negative evaluation of their social environment, and exhibit less behavioral problems. The child's age does not affect this relationship.

The child's birth rank. An effect of the child's birth rank on emotional reactions is only evident in the 8 to 16 year olds' experience of family relations. Univariate variance analysis showed that children who are an only child experience more negative feelings towards the father ($F=3.92$, $p<.05$) and also more positive feelings towards the father ($F=3.34$, $p<.05$). However, one should not attach too much importance to these results. First of all, this is probably a test artefact of the Family Relations Test (when items cannot be attributed to siblings, which is the case with an only child, the chance is greater that they will be attributed to the parents). Moreover, the number of 8 to 16 year old children who are an only child is very low in our study (n=5).

Disease characteristics

The correlations between the disease variables and emotion variables for children are reported in Appendix VII. Data on the disease characteristics are presented in Appendix I. The significant relationships are discussed below, by disease characteristic.

Time since diagnosis. Time since diagnosis refers to the time which has passed since cancer was diagnosed in the child. It tells us nothing about the duration of the child's disease symptoms. Our group is composed in such a way that the time since the children's diagnosis is 4 months, 1 year, 2 years, or 3-3 $1/2$ years. There is one anxiety variable which is significantly related to the time since diagnosis. As the time since diagnosis increases, the 4 to 12 year old children become blocked less often during the hospital play. The remaining anxiety measures, including the parents' assessment of the child's anxiety, are not significantly related to the time since diagnosis. In the 4 to 12 year old group, the children project more positive feelings during the hospital play as the time since diagnosis increases. For the 8 to 16 year olds, negative self-esteem increases as the disease has been diagnosed longer ago. The fathers judge their child (in all age groups) to be more depressed as the time since diagnosis increases. This relationship is not evident in the mothers' assessment, nor is there a significant relationship between the other depression measures of the child and time since diagnosis. The experience of family relations only appears to have a significant relationship with the time since diagnosis for the younger children (4-7 years). They experience more negative feelings towards siblings as the time since diagnosis increases.

The prognosis. The prognosis has been assessed by the pediatrician as good for 60% of the children and as poor for 40% of the children. The survival chances of the child with a good prognosis have been estimated at 50% and the survival chances with a poor prognosis have been estimated lower. Only the variable concerning the child's experience of family relations shows a significant relationship with the prognosis. The 4 to 7 year old children experience more positive and less negative feelings towards siblings if the child's prognosis is poor. The 8 to 16 year olds, on the other hand, experience more negative feelings towards the mother if the prognosis is poor.

The diagnosis. The children have been divided into groups, according to the type of diagnosis: a group of children with leukemia (23%) and a group of children with tumors (77%). The latter group also includes children with Morbus Hodgkin and lymphosarcoma. The 4 to 12 year old children with leukemia project more fear of pain and procedures and more feelings of loneliness and isolation. Children with leukemia (in all age groups) have more sleeping problems, but only according to the fathers' assessment. The greater fear of pain and procedures among children with leukemia is probably caused by the fact that these children are regularly subjected to painful procedures such as bone marrow aspirations and lumbar punctures.

A relapse or recurrence. Children in the 4 to 12 year old group who have or have had a relapse of leukemia or a recurrence of the tumor, project more fear of pain and procedures and more feelings of loneliness and isolation. The mothers report more problems at school for children who have or have had a relapse or recurrence. There is a relationship between a relapse or recurrence and feelings of pessimism in the older children (13-16 years). As a result of the small sample size of this age group, however, the correlation is not significant.

First remission. Children in the 4 to 12 year old group who are still in continous first remission at the time of the study, i.e. those for whom the disease has been successfully treated and for whom the symptoms have not returned again, project less fear of pain and procedures and less feelings of loneliness and isolation. The mothers report less problems at school for children who are in their first remission.

In (subsequent) remission. Children who are in continuous first remission or in subsequent remission at the time of the study are assessed by their mother to be more open and less introvert. The mothers also report less problems at school for these children.

Treatment duration. As the treatment is or has been more prolonged, the 4 to 12 year old children project more feelings of loneliness and isolation, but more positive feelings too. As the treatment takes or has taken more time, the negative self-esteem increases in the 8 to 16 year old children. The fathers assess their child as less cheerful and more depressed in the case of a longer treatment period. Fathers also report more sleeping problems and more problems at school for the child. Only the latter is reported by the mothers as well. The young children (4-7 years) experience more negative feelings towards siblings as the treatment duration increases, while the older children (8-16 years) experience more negative feelings towards the mother.

Undergoing treatment. The 4 to 12 year old children project more fear of pain and procedures and more feelings of loneliness and isolation if they are still undergoing treatment at the time of the study. The mothers report more problems at school and the fathers report more eating problems for the children if the children are still undergoing treatment.

Frequency of visits to the clinic. The 4 to 12 year old children project more fear of pain and procedures, more feelings of loneliness and isolation, and more feelings of grief as they have to go to the clinic more often for outpatient treatment and/or checkups at the time of the study. The 8 to 16 year old children describe themselves as less anxious, but show signs of greater tension during the interview (longer latency) as the frequency of visits to the clinic increases. The young children (4-7 years) experience less negative feelings and more positive feelings towards siblings as they have to go to the clinic more often, while the older children (8-16 years) experience less negative feelings towards the father. Finally, the mothers report more problems at school for children who have to go to the clinic often for treatment and/or checkups.

Number of hospital admissions. As the child has been admitted to hospital more often, the 8 to 16 year old children show signs of greater tension during the interview (longer latency). The 4 to 12 year old children project more positive feelings in the hospital play as they have been admitted to hospital more often. The higher the number of hospital admissions, the more negative feelings the 8 to 16 year old children have towards the mother, and the more positive feelings they have towards the father. Mothers report more bedwetting for children who have had more hospital admissions.

Number of days in hospital. The 4 to 12 year old children project more feelings of frustration in the hospital play as the number of days spent in hospital increases. For the 8 to 16 year old children, the negative feelings towards the mother increases as the number of days spent in hospital increases. Fathers report more bed-wetting for children who have spent more days in hospital.

Physical-visible consequences. As more physical restrictions and visible disfigurements (amputation, baldness, etc.) result from the disease and/or treatment, the 4 to 12 year old children become blocked more often during the hospital play and project less positive feelings during this play. The young children (4-7 years) experience less negative feelings towards siblings as the physical-visible effects are more evident. Mothers more often report bed-wetting and problems at school for children who have more physical-visible impairments resulting from the disease and/or treatment.

This summary may create the impression that disease characteristics have an important influence on the child's emotional reactions, however, this is only true in a limited sense. Most of the child's anxiety and depression measures are not influenced at all or only affected by a few disease characteristics. Only among the 4 to 12 year olds do we see a clear influence of various disease characteristics on the fear of pain and procedures and on the feelings of loneliness and isolation. Among the older children there is an influence on the child's self-esteem (8-12 years). Some influence of disease characteristics can be seen from the way the child experiences family relations. This reveals itself in the feelings of young children towards siblings and in the feelings of older children towards the mother. With regard to behavioral problems, the influence is most evident in the child's problems at school as reported by the mother. The child's motivation for and pleasure in attending school, and school absenteeism not caused by physical condition, are clearly influenced by the disease and treatment conditions of the child.

A small number of disease characteristics affect both the communication style of the parents and the emotional reactions of the child. For this reason, partial correlations have been performed to examine the extent to which the relationships we found continue to exist between the parents' communication style and the child's emotional reactions, after this effect of disease characteristics has been removed. As already noted in section 6.1, disease characteristics do not appear to alter the relationships found between the communication style and emotional reactions (the partial correlations are almost equal to the correlations).

The influence of biographical and disease characteristics on the parents' emotional reactions

Biographical characteristics

The parent's sex. The emotional reactions of the parents appear to be clearly related to the parent's sex. The significant correlations between sex and emotion variables are presented in Table 8.2.5. Compared with the fathers, the mothers report more psychological and psychosomatic stress reactions and more anxiety during the interview. Moreover, they consult their family doctor more often for their own complaints. As for the remaining emotion variables, including the projection of feelings specifically associated with the situation created by the disease, mothers score somewhat higher than fathers, but this difference is not significant.

The sex-determined differences between the parents correspond with the psychometric data of the instruments (Wilde, 1970; Ormel, 1980a; Van der Ploeg et al., 1980). Women generally score higher on questionnaires measuring unpleasant emotions. The above-mentioned sex-determined differences are the reason why the statistical tests have been performed separately for the mothers and the fathers.

Table 8.2.5
Pearson correlations (r) between sex and several emotion variables of the parents (n=159).

Emotion variables of the parents	**Sex of the parent** r
Psychological stress reactions (W-P)	.34**
Psychosomatic stress reactions (W-PS)	.29**
Anxiety-state (SRQ-AS)	.23*
Frequency of visits to the doctor (MC-D)	.24*

* = $p<.05$
** = $p<.01$

The parent's age. The parent's age does not show any relationship with the parents' emotional reactions, neither for mothers nor fathers.

The education of the parents. The education of the parents has a few significant correlations with the parents' projection of feelings specifically related to the situation created by the disease. These correlations are presented in Table 8.2.6.

As the mothers' educational level increases, the mothers project more feelings of anxiety and insecurity, more anxiety about not being able to keep it up, and more feelings of guilt about the child's disease. The same relationships are found for fathers, except for feelings of guilt. Moreover, fathers with a higher level of education project less

Table 8.2.6
Pearson correlations (r) between education and several emotion variables of the mothers (n=81) and fathers (n=78).

Emotion variables of the parents	Education of the mothers r	fathers r
Projective measures:		
Anxiety and insecurity (IBP-AI)	.30**	.23*
Anxiety about not being able to keep it up (IBP-AK)	.23*	.26*
Feelings of guilt (IBP-G)	.30**	.11
Positive feelings (IBP-P)	-.01	-.39**

* = $p<.05$
** = $p<.01$

positive feelings. No significant relationship with the parents' education can be found for the direct measures of anxiety and stress reactions, a finding which corresponds with the psychometric data on the questionnaires (Ormel, 1980a; Van der Ploeg et al., 1980).

The socio-economic status of the parents. The socio-economic status of the parents only correlates significantly with the fathers' projection of positive feelings (r=-.36, p<.01). As the socio-economic status is higher, the fathers project less positive feelings. No relationship with the parents' socio-economic status is found for the remaining emotion variables.

Disease characteristics

The correlations between the disease variables of the child and the emotion variables of the parents are presented in Appendix VII. The significant relationships are discussed below, by disease characteristic.

Time since diagnosis. As the time since the child's diagnosis increases, mothers project more feelings of loneliness and isolation and fathers report more psychosomatic stress reactions.

The prognosis. A good or a poor prognosis for the child (as assessed by the pediatrician) is not significantly related to emotional reactions, neither for the mothers nor the fathers.

The diagnosis. Mothers of children with leukemia are more pessimistic about the course of their child's illness than mothers of children with a solid tumor. This relationship is not found among the fathers.

Relapse or recurrence. As children have or have had a relapse or recurrence, both mothers and fathers are more pessimistic about the course of their child's illness. At the same time, the fathers project less anxiety about not being able to keep it up when the child has or has had a relapse or recurrence. Otherwise this disease characteristic is not significantly related to the emotional reactions of the parents.

First remission. If children are in continuous first remission the fathers are less pessimistic about the course of their child's illness, but they project more feelings of anxiety about not being able to keep it up. There is no significant relationship with the mothers' emotion variables.

In (subsequent) remission. If children are in first remission or are in subsequent remission after a relapse or recurrence, the fathers are less pessimistic about the course of their child's illness and they project more positive feelings. No influence of this disease characteristic is found among the mothers.

Treatment duration. As the child's treatment is or has been more prolonged, the mothers report more psychological and psychosomatic stress reactions. They are also more pessimistic about the course of their child's illness. The fathers report more anxiety during the interview as the child's treatment takes or has taken longer.

Undergoing treatment. If children have finished treatment, the mothers project more feelings of loneliness and isolation than mothers whose children are still undergoing treatment. The fathers of children whose treatment has been finished project more positive feelings than fathers whose children are still undergoing treatment.

Frequency of visits to the clinic. As the child has to go to the clinic more often for treatment and/or checkups at the time of the study, the fathers are more pessimistic about the course of their child's illness. No significant relationship has been found among the mothers.

Number of hospital admissions. As the child has been admitted more often into hospital, the mothers report more psychosomatic stress reactions. No significant relationship has been found among the fathers.

Number of days in hospital. As the child has spent more days in hospital, the mothers report more psychological and more psychosomatic stress reactions. This disease characteristic is not related to the emotion variables of the fathers.

Physical-visible consequences. As more physical restrictions and visible disfigurements result from the disease and/or treatment, the mothers project less feelings of loneliness and isolation and the fathers use more sleeping pills and sedatives.

The above discussion indicates that specific disease and treatment conditions of the child only have a limited influence on the parents' emotional reactions. On a number of emotion variables they have no influence at all. Moreover, the relationships found among the mothers and the fathers differ considerably from each other. Pessimism and thoughts of losing the child are most clearly influenced by the disease characteristics of the child. This is the case in both mothers and fathers. A certain influence of disease characteristics on feelings of loneliness and isolation only occurs among the mothers, and a prolonged clinical treatment of the child leads to more stress reactions, especially among the mothers. During the interview, some fathers mention their partner's heavier burden. For example, one father says:

> "I left too much up to her. My wife was at the hospital the whole day and I only came after work. And she always went to the clinic alone. A few weeks ago she just collapsed. Then you begin putting things in perspective. You

realize that it can't go on like this. Now I go along too and if they don't like it at work, then I'll just call in sick."

There are no biographical or disease characteristics which correlate with both the communication style and the emotion variables of the parent. As already mentioned in section 6.2, these cannot influence the relationships found between the communication style and the emotional reactions of the parent. This applies to both the relationships found for the mothers and to those found for the fathers.

8.3. The child's defensiveness and its relationship with the emotional reactions of the child and with the communication style of the parents

The degree of defensiveness in the 8 to 16 year old children has been measured with the defense scale (DESC). This questionnaire measures one aspect of defensiveness, namely the denial of anxieties and other unpleasant emotions and experiences every child has or has had sometimes. The defense scale enables us to examine whether children with cancer, when reacting to the situation which they are in, use a form of intrapsychological coping such as defense more extensively than healthy peers. Furthermore, we are able to determine whether the emotional reactions, which we have measured directly and indirectly, are influenced by the child's tendency to deny unpleasant emotions and experiences. Finally, we can test whether the communication style of the parents is related to the child's defensiveness. The number of significant correlations between the emotion variables and the defense variable turns out to be considerable and, on the whole, the correlations are quite high. Thus the relationship can be said to be quite strong. There are not as many significant correlations between the communication variables and the defense variable but, even so, they are greater than the 5% which can be expected on the basis of chance. However, the correlations between the last two variables are not very high so that there is only a weak relationship. The main results can be summarized as follows:

- Children with cancer between the ages of 8 and 12 years do not show a stronger tendency to deny anxieties and other unpleasant emotions and experiences than healthy peers.
- Children who have a stronger tendency to deny anxieties and other unpleasant emotions and experiences, describe themselves in the questionnaires (direct measures) as less anxious and less

depressed, report less negative expectations for the future, and show less negative self-esteem. On the indirect measures, the children project less diffuse anxiety and less feelings of pessimism as they are more defensive. Moreover, their latency is shorter but the number of blocks is greater.
- Children indicate that they experience less negative feelings towards their siblings and less positive feelings towards their mother as their defensiveness is stronger.
- Parents judge their child to be less depressed if the child's defensiveness is stronger.
- Parents communicate less with their child about his or her emotional experience as the child is more defensive. Otherwise the child's defensiveness does not play any role in the way the parents communicate with their child about the disease.

The results are explained further below.

The degree of the child's defensiveness

In order to compare the scores on the defense scale of the children with cancer to the scores of a group of healthy children, we only have data available from 366 boys and girls between the ages of 9 and 12 years (Klomp et al., 1979). The 8 to 12 year old group of children with cancer is the most eligible one for making a comparison. The mean scores of the 8 to 12 year olds do not deviate from the mean scores of this group of healthy peers. This means that a personality trait of defensiveness does not occur more often in children with cancer in this age group. We cannot rule out the possibility that children with cancer deny specific anxieties such as fear of death more often (see section 8.1), but there does not seem to be any generalization. There are also no indications that such a personality trait develops in the children over time. No relationship can be shown between defensiveness and time since diagnosis. Neither are disease characteristics, for example, the nature of the prognosis, related to defensiveness. The age and sex of the children does not influence defensiveness either. In Klomp et al.'s study, boys scored significantly higher on the defense scale than girls. This turns out not to be the case in our study. The boys with cancer score somewhat higher than the girls but the difference is not significant.

Besides a coping style or defense mechanism of denial, interview data show that children also use other defense mechanisms. We can see examples of this in the statements from the older children, who are more capable of reflecting on their own behavior. For example, a sixteen year old girl indicates how she could avoid reality for awhile:

> "When I went to the Emma Kinder Ziekenhuis they talked about a growth. Kind of strange but I just didn't think about it. During all those tests I just didn't know anything and I didn't ask anything. I didn't really want to know the kind of ward I was in and what was wrong with the other children. After a few weeks I saw my parents coming down the hall and I walked cheerfully towards them but they had just been told the test results by the doctor. Then I asked them if it was serious and they started to cry right away and said I had bone cancer. Then we all cried."

Attempts by the children to control the situation by using intellectualization are also evident. A thirteen year old girl says:

> "There was a chance that my leg would have to be amputated during the operation. This really worried me for awhile. Then I kept asking the doctor about the chances that my leg would not be amputated and I asked a lot about a prosthesis. Whether I'd be able to play hockey and run with one of those. Because then you certainly start to think about life and what it would be like with a prosthesis. The doctor told me about the options and showed me photographs. For the rest, we stuck to the treatment schedule. Then you knew what you had to do."

Behavior that can be seen as reaction formation also occurs, such as being overly cheerful, brave, and tough. A fifteen year old girl relates:

> "I was in hospital for treatment at Christmas too. I was very ill and laid there throwing up all the time and it was very hard on my father and mother. Then I decided to cheer them up and began to sing: "Always look on the bright side of life". Well that wasn't such a good idea. Then my mother was really upset."

The relationship between defensiveness and emotional reactions of the child

The defense scale correlates negatively with a large number of anxiety and depression variables and many correlations are significant. These are presented in Appendix III. As the 8 to 16 year old children show a stronger tendency to deny anxieties and other unpleasant emotions and experiences which every child has or has had sometimes, they describe themselves as less anxious (anxiety trait) and less depressed and report less negative self-esteem and less negative expectations for the future. All of these relationships are significant. The emotional behavior of the child assessed by the parents is significantly related to the child's defensiveness on one point. As the 8 to 16 year old children react more defensively, the parents (both mothers and fathers) judge them to be less depressed. The assumption of the projective measures of the children's emotional reactions being much less influenced by defensiveness than the direct measures (self-reports) turns out to be incorrect. Just like the direct measures, reasonably high negative correlations are also found in the case of the projective measures. As defensiveness is stronger, the 8 to 12 year old children project significantly less diffuse anxiety in the hospital play and the 13 to 16 year old children project significantly less feelings of pessimism. The results on latency and blocks are contradictory. A slight but significant negative correlation is found between the defense scale and latency in the interview, but this does not happen to be the case in the hospital play. Conversely, a reasonably high positive correlation is found between the defense scale and the number of blocks in the hospital play, but this is not found in the interview. As defensiveness is stronger, the 8 to 16 year old children have a shorter latency in the interview and the 8 to 12 year old children have more blocks in the hospital play. This means that children having a stronger defense reaction become blocked more often during the play, in which they are reminded of unpleasant emotions and experiences. However, they give a quicker - and, as far as the interviewer could determine, an evasive and negative - answer to questions about their illness and other emotionally-charged topics during the interview. Finally, the child's defensiveness shows a few weak but significant relationships with the child's experience of family relations. As defensiveness is stronger in the 8 to 16 year old children, they indicate that they experience less negative feelings towards siblings and less positive feelings towards the mother. The latter is remarkable because defensiveness, or a tendency to deny negative emotions, seems to influence the experience of positive feelings as well.

The above findings indicate that one should not assume, as a matter of course, that children who describe themselves as not very anxious and not very depressed, and who project few feelings of anxiety and depression, are indeed not very anxious and depressed. We may assume that a number of children use an intrapsychological coping style or defense mechanism, thus denying their feelings of anxiety and depression. When testing the relationship between the communication style of the parents and the emotional reactions of the child, we have taken this finding into account (see section 6.1).

The relationship between the parents' communication style and the child's defensiveness

On the whole, the correlations between the communication variables of the parents (communication style of one or both parents) and the defense scale of the child appear to be low and negative (see Appendix III). There is one significant correlation. As the child is more defensive, the parents communicate less with the child about his or her emotional experience. The relationship is not strong but does correspond with what parents state in the interview (see section 7.7). They say that a reason for them not to ask the child about worries or grief is that the child always reacts defensively or always denies worries and grief. We conclude from these findings that the child's defensiveness only plays a minor role in the parents' communication with their child about the disease.

8.4. The relationship of the communication style with the coping style and the child-rearing attitudes of the parents

We have examined whether the parents' communication style is strongly related to the parents' personality traits. If so, the parents' communication style should be considered difficult to influence. These personality traits concern the parents' coping style (how problems are generally handled) and child-rearing attitudes. Using the Utrecht Coping List (UCL), seven coping styles have been measured. Moreover, four different child-rearing attitudes have been measured using the Amsterdam version of the Parental Attitude Research Instrument (A-PARI). For both mothers and fathers, the communication style appears to be related to some extent to their coping style. The number of significant correlations for both is greater than the 5% expected on the basis of chance, but the pattern of correlations is different. Only the mothers' communication style is slightly related to their child-rearing attitudes. The number of significant correlations for the fathers is lower than the 5% expected on the basis of chance. On the whole, the correlations are not very high which means that the relationships are weak. Before presenting the results in more detail, they can be summarized as follows:

- Mothers having a coping style of active problem-solving talk more often with their child about the disease.
- Fathers having a coping style of active problem-solving have given their child more information about the diagnosis and prognosis at an early stage.
- Mothers having a coping style of seeking social support express their grief to the child more often.
- Fathers having a coping style of seeking social support have given their child more information about the prognosis at an early stage, more often express their grief to the child, and talk with their child about the disease more often.
- Mothers having a coping style of a depressive reaction pattern express their grief to the child more often.
- Fathers having a coping style of comforting cognitions have given their child more information about the prognosis at an early stage.
- Mothers having an over-protective child-rearing attitude communicate less with their child about his or her emotional experience, express their worry to the child less often, and talk to the child about the disease less often.
- Mothers having a stronger autocratic child-rearing attitude express their worries to the child less often and talk to their child about the disease less often.
- Mothers having a stronger autonomy-promoting child-rearing attitude have given their child less information about the diagnosis or have given information at a later stage.

The findings are presented in more detail below.

The relationship between communication style and coping style of the parents

A coping style of avoidance and a wait-and-see attitude, a coping style of palliative actions, and a coping style of expression of emotions/anger are not related in any way to the communication style, neither for mothers nor for fathers. It is most surprising that parents accustomed to a strategy of avoidance when encountering problems do not exhibit this behavior when it involves informing the child about the disease. They have not given their child less information about the diagnosis and prognosis or given information at a later stage. There are a few significant relationships between the other coping styles and the communication style. These are presented in Table 8.4.1 and Table 8.4.2.

There appears to be little correspondence between the findings

Table 8.4.1
Pearson correlations (r) between the coping variables "Active problem-solving" and "Seeking social support", on the one hand, and communication variables (CSP) of the mothers (n=81) and fathers (n=78), on the other hand.

Communication variables	Coping variables			
	Active problem-solving		Seeking social support	
	Mothers r	Fathers r	Mothers r	Fathers r
Information about the diagnosis	-.04	.27*	.04	-.01
Information about the prognosis	.12	.35**	.01	.25*
Expression of grief	.03	.11	.32**	.32**
Communication about the disease at the child's initiative	.25*	.02	.17	.26*
Communication about the disease at the parent's initiative	-.08	.01	-.01	.23*

* = p<.05
** = p<.01

for the mothers and those for the fathers. The relationship is only the same in the case of the coping style of seeking social support and the expression of grief. As mothers and fathers seek more social support, they express their grief to the child more often. Otherwise the relationships for mothers and fathers are different. As fathers deal with problems more actively, they have already given their child more information about the diagnosis and prognosis in the initial stage of the disease. This relationship is conceivable because informing the child can be seen as a first step in dealing with a problem, namely defining the problem. However, this relationship does not occur among the mothers, as their coping style is related to a different aspect of communication with the child. As mothers more actively deal with problems, the child takes the initiative more often to talk with the mother about the disease in the current stage. As previously mentioned, the coping style *seeking social support* has only one corresponding result among the mothers and the fathers. As mothers and fathers seek more social sup-

Table 8.4.2
Pearson correlations (r) between the coping variables "Depressive reaction pattern" and "Comforting cognitions", on the one hand, and communication variables (CSP) of the mothers (n=81) and fathers (n=78), on the other hand.

	Coping variables			
	Depressive reaction pattern		Comforting cognitions	
	Mothers	Fathers	Mothers	Fathers
Communication variables	r	r	r	r
Information about the prognosis	.04	.11	.03	.26*
Expression of grief	.26*	.07	.07	.06

* = p<.05

port, they express their grief to the child more often. Among the fathers, seeking more social support is also associated with giving the child more information about the prognosis at an early stage, and with more communication between father and child in the current stage of the disease, both at the child's initiative and at the father's own initiative.

In Table 8.4.2 we can also see that mothers with a more depressive reaction pattern express their grief to the child more often. Fathers who cope with problems by having more reassuring and comforting thoughts have given their child more information about the prognosis at an early stage. We can conclude from these findings that there is a certain relationship between coping style and communication style, especially among the fathers. However, as the correlations are not high, this is a rather weak relationship.

The relationship between communication style and child-rearing attitudes of the parents

Significant relationships between communication style and child-rearing attitudes are only found for the mothers and are presented in Table 8.4.3.

As the mothers have a stronger over-protective attitude towards child-rearing, they communicate less with their child about his or her emotional experience, they express their worries less often to the child, and the child takes the initiative less often to talk about the disease with the mother in the current stage. In the previous

Table 8.4.3
Pearson correlations (r) between child-rearing attitude scales and communication variables (CSP) for the mothers (n=81).

	Child-rearing attitude scales		
	Over-protective attitude	Autocratic attitude	Autonomy-promoting attitude
Communication variables:	r	r	r
Information about the diagnosis	-.15	-.20	-.30**
Communication about the child's emotional experience	-.23*	-.10	.19
Expression of worries	-.34**	-.29**	-.22
Communication about the disease at the child's initiative	-.33**	-.35**	-.10

* = $p<.05$
** = $p<.01$

sections, the phenomenon of mutual protection has been discussed several times. This phenomenon seems to occur here as well. Mothers who tend to protect their child from problems, avoid arousing negative emotions in the child by asking less about the child's emotional experience of the illness, and avoid burdening the child with their own worries. In turn, the child protects the mother by hardly ever discussing the disease. By the way, this phenomenon does not occur among the fathers. The reason for this is unclear. It cannot be attributed to a difference in communication style, nor to a difference in child-rearing attitudes between the group of mothers and the group of fathers. The parent's sex does not play a role in the child-rearing attitudes. Mothers express their worries less often to the child and the child takes the initiative less often to talk with the mother about the disease, not only in the case of a stronger over-protective child-rearing attitude, but also in the case of a stronger autocratic child-rearing attitude. The negative correlation between an autonomy-promoting attitude and information about the diagnosis is surprising. Mothers with a stronger autonomy-promoting child-rearing attitude, have given their child information at a later stage and/or less information about the diagnosis. This seems to contradict with a child-rearing attitude which is intended to promote the child's independence. An over-protective or an autocratic child-rearing attitude would sooner be associated with giving less information about the disease to the child. But this does not turn out to be the case. For that matter, the correlations are not high here either. Therefore the relationship between child-rearing attitudes and communication style of the mothers should be qualified as weak.

9. Conclusions

The concept of open communication, conceived to be a unidimensional concept in the literature, does not appear to exist as such. From our study, open communication emerges as a multidimensional concept. The way in which the child is informed about the disease, for example, does not predict the transfer of information about emotions or the extent to which child and parents communicate about the illness. The wide range of emotional reactions we studied in children and parents could not be reduced to a unidimensional concept of negative emotions either. For this reason, our hypothesis that an open communication style is associated with less negative emotions and more positive emotions has been tested for each variable separately.

In our study, giving information as a part of open communication is related to the child's emotional reactions. Children who have been informed by their parents about the diagnosis and prognosis at an early stage are less anxious, less depressed, have a less negative evaluation of their social environment, and exhibit less behavioral problems than children who have been informed by their parents at a later stage or hardly at all. This finding applies to children of all ages from the age of four and above. We think it is justified to speak of a favorable effect of open information on the child's emotional experience. After all, the information has been given in the past, while the child's emotional reactions have been determined in the present. Therefore it is impossible that the child's emotional reactions should reversely influence the information provided by the parents, unless we assume that the child's emotional reactions are a stable personality trait, which would have already determined the information at the moment it was given by the parents. However, we do not find any indication that this might be the case. Parents who have given their child little information about the disease explain their behavior by saying they think the child is still too young or they don't want to burden the child with such serious facts. None of the parents mention their child's anxiety or depression as a reason for withholding information. Learning the diagnosis is obviously a painful affair for children. Yet none of the children declare they would have preferred the parents or doctors, who gave them this information, to have remained silent about the facts. Children who were informed about the disease by their parents at an early stage experience a greater availability of sources of information and less obstacles to information. These children are less anxious, less depressed, have a less negative self-image, and exhibit fewer behavioral problems.

An important argument for fully informing children about the disease at an early stage is based on our finding that at least one-third of the children had been bluntly informed about the disease by fellow patients or peers in the home environment. Thus we see that attempts at controlling the flow of information fail in many cases. Our finding that open information to the child results in the child being less anxious and less depressed, corresponds with previously conducted research. We also found support for Spinetta's (1980) view that a child loses confidence if information about the disease is withheld. Children in our study who have not received much information about their illness or did not receive this information until later, have a more negative opinion about their social environment. Just like Koocher and O'Malley (1981) and Márky (1982), we found a marked discrepancy between the parents' reports of the information that was given to the child and the children's reports. Although a high correspondence exists between the child's knowledge about the illness and the information the parents report to have given the child, the children named their parents to a much lesser degree as the source of their knowledge. We assume this to indicate that the children already understood the nature of their disease before the parents informed them.

The relationship between informing the child and the emotional reactions of the parents is more equivocal. We could not find any relationship among the mothers. Among the fathers, on the contrary, open information is associated with more negative emotions in the current stage of the illness. It is not clear whether we should call it an effect of information on emotions. The argument in favor of calling it an effect is the same as in the case of the children: information has been given in the past, while the emotional reactions have been determined in the present. It is possible that anxiety, insecurity, and feelings of helplessness were already present in the past as dispositions. It is not very likely, however, that such dispositions should stimulate parents to give information to the child. If we should call it an effect of information on the emotional reactions of the fathers, then it is remarkable that this negative effect does not occur among the mothers. One possible explanation for this difference may be that the fathers' way of informing the child is associated with a coping style of active problem-solving. This does not apply to the mothers. Fathers who informed their child about the disease at an early stage are characterized by a coping style of actively dealing with problems. We postulated that information about the disease, among other things, aids primary control of the situation. By giving information, one enables the child to define the situation, which is a first step towards solving the problem. Fathers who have a coping style of actively dealing with problems probably experience more negative emotions when it becomes apparent that their possibilities of primary control do not go beyond defining the problem. Data in the literature indicate this kind of relationship between coping style and emotional reactions. Persons who have a strong commitment to control situations, become very upset and desperate when their attempts to control the situation appear to be in vain (Glass, 1977a, 1977b).

It is suggested in the literature that creating an atmosphere in which children feel free to talk about their worries and fears is good for the child's emotional experience. In our study we asked parents whether they actively encouraged their child to express his or her worries and grief. A considerable number of parents never asked the child about his or her emotional experience of the illness. We did not find a relationship between the children's emotional reactions and this aspect of the parental communication style. We also considered the parent's expression of worries and grief to their child to be part of communication about the emotional experience. Many parents hide their worries and grief from the child, but we could not find a relationship here either between the child's emotional reactions and this part of the parental communication style. There seems to be no need for parents to pretend they are cheerful which, by the way, does not mean that children confronted too often with their parents' worries and grief would not experience it as a burden. After all, we noticed that many children try to control the emotions of their parents and their own emotions. Protecting the parents and protecting themselves seems to be an important motive for the children. From the behavior of parents who never ask the child about his or her worries and grief, and who never express their own worries and grief to the child, it can be inferred that they also have a need to protect themselves and the child.

A relationship between communication about the emotional experience and the emotional reactions of the parents could only be demonstrated for the mothers. Mothers who actively ask about the child's emotional experience appear to have more feelings of loneliness and isolation. Mothers who sometimes express their worries to the child exhibit more psychological stress reactions and more feelings of helplessness. This indicates that asking about the child's emotional experience and expressing emotions to the child, either increase the mothers' negative emotions or are signs of diminished control of one's own emotions when the intensity of emotions increases. A similar phenomenon occurs among the children, but this involves the frequency of their taking the initiative to talk with their parents about the illness. They take the initiative more often as they experience more feelings of grief and pessimism, and as they exhibit more behavioral problems. We assume these emotions to be the reason for communication about the illness. After all, should the child experience talking about the disease as too great a burden, it would just stop taking the initiative to do so. Moreover, the children are generally content with the frequency of their talks with their parents about the illness and they want to determine themselves how often, and in what manner, they will discuss the disease.

Neither the frequency of parents taking the initiative to talk with their child about the disease nor their talking freely about the disease with others in the presence of the child, have an unequivocal relationship with the children's emotional reactions. Some negative emotions are stronger while other negative emotions are actually weaker when parents take the initiative more often to talk with their child about the disease and talk freely with others in the presence of the child. We do not have a clear explanation for this finding. On the one hand, feelings of anxiety, frustration, and pessimism increase in the children when they are regularly confronted with their illness by the conversations taking place "above their heads". On the other hand, it seems to arouse the child's suspicions if parents are careful with what they tell others about the disease in the presence of the child. Communication about the disease in the current stage of the illness does not have any relationship with the fathers' emotional reactions, and only in a very limited sense with the mothers'.

From the above, we can draw the conclusion that our study confirms the assumption in the literature of open information having a favorable effect on the child's emotional experience. Our research results correspond with the infrequent empirical research conducted in this area (Koocher & O'Malley, 1981; Spinetta & Maloney, 1978). As for the parents, however, our findings are contradictory to previously conducted research. This only concerns one single study though by Spinetta et al. (1981) conducted among parents whose child had died. Our study does not support the assumption that open communication about the emotional experience of the illness and open communication about the disease during the entire course of the illness has a favorable influence on the emotional experience of children and parents.

Using information obtained about the disease, the child is able to understand the situation better, increasing the feeling of control and motivating the child to cooperate with the treatment. Open information can reduce the child's anxiety, depression, and behavioral problems, but cannot remove them. Children with cancer who could be compared with healthy peers, i.e. the 8 to 12 year old children, appeared to be more anxious and more depressed and had a more negative self-image. A comparison with healthy peers was not possible for the younger and older children. However, from a comparison amongst the children with cancer, especially the younger children turned out to be more anxious and depressed. This corresponds with the findings of other researchers who found a markedly increased anxiety in younger children with cancer (Spinetta et al., 1973; Waechter, 1971), but did not find increased anxiety or a more negative self-image among adolescents (Kellerman et al., 1980; Zeltzer et al., 1980). In the literature, the low level of anxiety in adolescents is attributed to the development of effective coping strategies, including denial. Nevertheless, we found that adolescents do not deny anxieties and other unpleasant emotions and experiences more strongly than younger children. Younger children, in turn, did not show stronger denial than healthy peers. We also found no evidence of adolescents denying their disease or the possible implications of their disease more strongly than younger children. Presumably the differences in intensity of emotions stem from the information which older children have received. After all, we found that older children are more fully informed about their illness already in the initial stage.

A surprising finding in our study is that parents of children with cancer do not have more psychological and psychosomatic stress reactions and do not experience any more anxiety than persons representing an average of the Dutch population. There is no difference in the parents' use of sleeping pills and sedatives or the frequency of visits to the doctor for their own complaints either. These findings contrast with data in the literature, which show more anxiety and depression in parents of children with cancer (Magni et al., 1983; Maguire, 1983; Powazek et al., 1980). Our findings do correspond with the conclusions of Kupst et al. (1982) and Márky (1982): most parents of children with cancer show an adequate adjustment to the illness and do not experience a prolonged disruption of their emotional balance. We too could observe that most parents are optimistic about the chances of a cure for their child, and although they do not completely deny the thought of possibly losing their child, they are capable of pushing these thoughts to the background. Despite a predominant optimism about a favorable outcome of the illness, and despite a 'normal' intensity of psychological and psychosomatic stress reactions and non-specific anxiety, parents do project more situation-specific emotions of anxiety and insecurity and feelings of helplessness. On the one hand, this could indicate that anxiety and uncertainty about the outcome of the illness and feelings of helplessness arising from a lack of control over the situation do not generalize to an overall decrease in well-being. On the other hand, it might be an indication of the effects of defense mechanisms. Parents deny their own negative emotions, but do project these onto others.

Besides negative feelings, many parents associate positive feelings as well with the situation created by the illness. These positive feelings clearly express a shift in values which occurs during the course of the illness. Just like in the study by Koocher and O'Malley (1981), a great number of parents in our study expressed their feeling that the family has grown closer together.

Differences in disease and treatment conditions of the children appear to have a very limited influence on the communication style, on the one hand, and on the emotional experience of children and parents, on the other hand. From this we conclude that the entire situational context, determined by the child's cancer, has a stronger influence than specific disease and treatment conditions. However, we did find a negative effect of time since diagnosis and treatment duration on the children's self-image. Negative self-esteem increases in the children as they have been diagnosed longer ago, and the treatment takes or has taken longer. If the treatment is more prolonged, the child experiences a diminished physical and social functioning and also a change in appearance over a longer period of time, which can harm the child's self-image. Stigmatization by the environment can negatively influence the child's self-image as well (Goffman, 1963).

Only among the mothers does protracted clinical treatment of the child lead to more psychological and psychosomatic stress reactions. Mothers generally have a larger part in caring for the child, also during clinical treatment. Consequently, they apparently experience a greater emotional burden than the fathers who, as suggested in the literature, find some distraction in their job (Cook, 1984; Koocher & O'Malley, 1981; Márky, 1982).

Only a slight relationship could be demonstrated between the communication style of the parents and their coping style and child-rearing attitudes. From this finding we draw the following conclusion: we do not expect such relatively stable personality traits as coping style or child-rearing attitudes to interfere with interventions to alter the parents' behavior with regard to communication style.

Open information and the law of double protection

Emotions such as the children's anxiety and depression and the parents' anxiety and helplessness can be attributed to prolonged uncertainty and limited control of the situation in which the children with cancer and their parents find themselves. Communication between child and parents consists to a large extent of attempts to reduce uncertainty and to increase control. Information about the disease can reduce the child's uncertainty. It enables the child to distinguish more properly between events which are threatening and events which are not. It provides the child with a safety signal and is an important means of achieving primary and secondary control of the situation. It motivates the child to make an (ongoing) effort to endure the highly aversive treatment. Moreover, understanding what is wrong with you can in itself provide some sense of control. However, knowing and understanding the facts, given the nature of the situation, is not enough for setting up an effective barrier against the threat. Thus most of the communication concentrates on protection from the arousal of negative emotions evoked by the threat. In the communication between child and parents, it is very striking that protecting oneself is often achieved through protecting the other. Attempts to influence the other person's appraisal in order to reduce the other person's negative emotions not only involve showing compassion and empathy, but also serve to protect oneself against confrontation with the other person's emotions. We call this the law of double protection. It is essential for the child to believe that his or her parents are strong: if they can handle the situation, it constitutes the signal that the threat can be averted. The parents, in turn, need to believe that the child is strong: if the child can handle the situation, it boosts their confidence that the child will survive. All attempts by the parents to conceal the true meaning of the situation from the child are attempts neither to burden nor to weaken the child. The parents avoidance of discussing his or her worries and grief related to the illness prevents the child from thinking about it, and protects the parents from being confronted with the child's emotions. Not only the parents achieve self-protection through the other person. The child achieves it as well. Not asking questions which might worry the parents, hiding grief, and being brave are attempts at preventing the parents from becoming distressed, and themselves from becoming overwhelmed by the parents' emotions. In order to be able to count their child among the lucky ones who will survive the disease, the parents create an image of vitality and zest for life. The striking attribution of properties to the child such as optimism, happiness, and cheerfulness - attributions which do not correspond with the child's actual emotional experience - is a form of illusory control, necessary to be able to keep on believing that fate will be kind to them.

In our opinion, the results of our study can be generalized to children with other life-threatening diseases. Therefore, on the basis of our research, we would like to make the following recommendations for a clinical policy regarding communication with a seriously ill child. Immediately after the child has been diagnosed, it is important to advise the parents to tell the child, as soon as possible, about the nature and possible implications of the disease. The doctor may offer his or her support to the parents and inform the child in the presence of the parents. If this information is passed on to the child right after the diagnosis, it can be combined with a message of hope. After all, emphasizing hope is realistic when explaining the possibilities for treatment to the child. This advice will certainly encounter resistance among some parents because these parents are afraid this information would burden their child too much. They are afraid that their child's reaction will be highly emotional and the child will lose courage. It's important to understand these feelings, but the doctor can reassure the parents that openly informing their child should not have harmful effects, that it will not affect the child's motivation for treatment, but on the contrary keeping this information from the child will prove to be detrimental. Our opinion is that the doctor is not the only person who may give this advice to the parents, but is certainly the most obvious person. In our study we observed that the doctor performs an important model function in the communication about the disease between child and parents. In the cases in which the doctor had openly discussed cancer and the survival chances in the presence of the child, the parents in our study reported they had initially been shocked by this frankness. However, they had not noticed any harmful effects to their child and it had facilitated their own communication about the illness with the child. When the information to the child about the disease is incorporated in the doctor's protocol, the other hospital staff will have to help the child assimilate this information, and to support the child and parents in their attempts to gain psychological control of their situation. It is important to leave it up to the child how often he or she wants to discuss the illness and his or her emotional experience. The child should not be forced to talk about it, but the often subtle hints which children give when they want to talk about the situation should be responded to. An area of tension exists between the need to control the situation through double protection, and the need to share thoughts and emotions with the other person. If the threatening stimuli and the emotions are too strong to be denied, then the need for sympathy and support becomes dominant. Open communication fulfills this need but does not mean that the operation of double protection has been ruled out. Concealing facts which cannot remain hidden from the child, strengthens the child's cognitions that "it's too bad to talk about". The child may draw the conclusion from this that his or her death is unavoidable. The child cannot distinguish between facts (a serious disease) and implications. The child accepts one of the possible implications - death - as an actual fact. Open information enables the child to discriminate between facts and the implications of facts. By supplying the facts and simultaneously offering reassurance and hope of a favorable outcome, the child will again be in a position to build up self-protection. Open information is a necessary condition for effective self-protection.

10. References

Ablin, A. R., Binger, C. M., Stein, R. C., Kushner, J. H., Zoger, S., & Mikkelson, C. (1971). A conference with the family of a leukemic child. *American Journal of Diseases of Children, 122,* 362-364.
Adams, M. A. (1978). Helping the parents of children with malignancy. *Journal of Pediatrics, 93,* 734-738.
Adams-Greenly, M. (1984). Helping children communicate about serious illness and death. *Journal of Psychosocial Oncology, 2*(2), 61-72.
Aken, M. A. van, Heezen, T. J., & Lieshout, C. F. van (1986). Beenmergpuncties bij kinderen met leukemie. Vaststelling en verlaging van pijn- en angstreacties. *Tijdschrift voor Kindergeneeskunde, 54,* 112-118.
Andrew, J. M. (1970). Recovery from surgery with and without preparatory instruction for three coping styles. *Journal of Personality and Social Psychology, 151,* 223-226.
Arnold, M. B. (1960). *Emotion and Personality* (2 vols.). New York: Columbia University Press.
Averill, J. R. (1973). Personal control over aversive stimuli and its relationship to stress. *Psychological Bulletin, 80,* 286-303.
Baarda, D. B., Londen, A. van, & Londen-Barentsen, W. M. (1983). *Handleiding (experimentele uitgave) Familie Relatie Test.* Lisse: Swets & Zeitlinger.
Bakker, F. C. (1981). *Persoonlijkheid en motorisch leren bij kinderen. Onderzoek naar de relatie van angst en struktureringstendentie met het leren mini-trampoline springen.* Academisch Proefschrift. Amsterdam: Academische Pers.
Bakker, F. C., & Wieringen, P. van (1985). Anxiety induced by ego and physical threat: Preliminary validation of a Dutch adaption of Spielberger's State-Trait Anxiety Inventory for Children (STAIC). In C. D. Spielberger, I. G. Sarason, & P. B. Defares (Eds.), *Stress and Anxiety* (Vol. 9, pp. 141-146). Washington: Hemisphere.
Bakker, H. D. (1982). Terminale zorg bij kinderen. *Nederlands Tijdschrift voor Geneeskunde, 126,* 720-724.
Barnlund, D. (1970). A transactional model of communication. In K. Sereno, & C. Mortensen (Eds.), *Foundations of communication theory* (pp. 83-102). New York: Harper & Row.
Bateson, G., Jackson, D. D., Haley, J., & Weakland, J. (1956). Toward a theory of schizophrenia. *Behavioral Science, 1,* 251-264.
Beakel, N. G., & Mehrabian, A. (1969). Inconsistent communications and psychopathology. *Journal of Abnormal Psychology, 74,* 126-130.
Bean, B. W. (1976). *An investigation of the reliability and validity of the family relations test.* Unpublished doctoral dissertation, University of Kansas. (University Microfilms No. 77-2188).
Beauchamp, N. F. (1974). The young child's perception of death (Doctoral dissertation 1974). *Dissertation Abstracts International, 35,* 6a.
Behrendt, H. (1980). Leukemie bij kinderen. *Para Medica,* (7), 17-22.
Behrendt, H. (1984). De prognose van acute lymfatische leukemie (ALL) bij kinderen. *Nederlands Tijdschrift voor Geneeskunde, 128,* 2138-2142.
Bene, E., & Anthony, J. (1978). *Manual for the children's version of the family relations test. An objective technique for exploring emotional attitudes in children* (rev. ed.). Windsor, England: NFER-Nelson.

Binger, C. M., Ablin, A. R., Feuerstein, R. C., Kushner, J. H., Zoger, S., & Mikkelsen, C. (1969). Childhood leukemia. Emotional impact on patient and family. *New England Journal of Medicine*, 280, 414-418.
Blom, J. E., Raymakers, M. J., Last, B. F., & Veldhuizen, A. M. van (1984). *Onderzoek naar het functioneren van het kind met een maligne aandoening op school*. Intern rapport. Kinderoncologisch Centrum te Amsterdam.
Bluebond-Langner, M. (1975). *Awareness and communication in terminally ill children: pattern, process, and pretense*. Unpublished doctoral dissertation, University of Illinois. (University Microfilms No. 76-6834).
Bluebond-Langner, M. (1977). Meanings of death to children. In H. Feifel (Ed.), *New meanings of death* (pp. 48-66). New York: McGraw-Hill.
Bonekamp, A. (1980). *Ouders van ernstig zieke en stervende kinderen. Opvoedings- en begeleidingsproblemen*. Meppel: Boom.
Boogaerts, M. A., & Dekker, A. W. (1983). Acute leukemie: behandeling en prognose. In K. Punt & R. L. Verwilghen (red.), *Acute leukemie* (pp. 50- 73). Alphen aan den Rijn: Stafleu.
Bowlby, J. (1973). *Attachment and loss: Vol. 2. Separation: Anxiety and Anger*. London: The Hogarth Press and the Institute of Psycho-Analysis.
Bozeman, M. F., Orbach, C. E., & Sutherland, A. M. (1955). Psychological impact of cancer and its treatment, III. The adaption of mothers to the threatened loss of their children through leukemia: Part I. *Cancer*, 8, 1- 19.
Bretherton, I., Fritz, J., Zahn-Waxler, C., & Ridgeway, D. (1986). Learning to talk about emotions: A functionalist perspective. *Child Development*, 57, 529-548.
Brewin, T. B. (1977). The cancer patient: communication and morale. *British Medical Journal*, 2, 1623-1627.
Brewster, A. B. (1982). Chronically ill hospitalized children's concepts of their illness. *Pediatrics*, 69, 355-362.
Breznitz, S. (1983). The seven kinds of denial. In S. Breznitz (Ed.), *The denial of stress* (pp. 257-280). New York: International Universities Press.
Brunnquell, D., & Hall, M. D. (1982). Issues in the psychological care of pediatric oncology patients. *American Journal of Orthopsychiatry*, 52, 32-44.
Burstein, S., & Meichenbaum, D. (1979). The work of worrying in children undergoing surgery. *Journal of Abnormal Child Psychology*, 7, 121-131.
Burton, L. (1975). *The family life of sick children. A study of families coping with chronic childhood disease*. London: Routledge & Kegan Paul.
Byrne, D. (1964). Repression-sensitization as a dimension of personality. In B. A. Maher (Ed.), *Progress in experimental personality research* (Vol. 1). New York: Academic Press.
Cairns, N. U., Clark, G. M., Smith, S. D., & Lansky, S. B. (1979). Adaptation of siblings to childhood malignancy. *Journal of Pediatrics*, 95, 484-487.
Cannel, C. F., & Kahn, R. L. (1953). The collection of data by interviewing. In L. Festinger & D. Katz (Eds.), *Research methods in the behavioral sciences* (pp. 327-380). New York: Dryden Press.
Centraal Bureau voor de Statistiek (CBS). (1980). *Leefsituatie-onderzoek*.
Childers, P., & Wimmer, M. (1971). The concept of death in early childhood. *Child Development*, 42, 1299-1301.
Chodoff, P., Friedman, S. B., & Hamburg, D. A. (1964). Stress, defenses and coping behavior: Observations in parents of children with malignant disease. *American Journal of Psychiatry*, 120, 743-749.
Cohen, S. (1980). Aftereffects of stress on human performance and social behavior: A review of research and theory. *Psychological Bulletin*, 88, 82-108.
Cohen, F., & Lazarus, R. S. (1973). Active coping processes, coping dispositions, and recovery from surgery. *Psychosomatic Medicine*, 35, 375-389.
Comaroff, J., & Maguire, P. (1981). Ambiguity and the search for meaning: Childhood leukaemia in the modern clinical context. *Social Science Medicine*, 15, 115-123.
Cook, J. A. (1984). Influence of gender on the problems of parents of fatally ill children. *Journal of Psychosocial Oncology*, 2(1), 71-91.
Cummings, E. M., Zahn-Waxler, A., & Radke-Yarrow, M. (1981). Young children's re-

sponses to expressions of anger and affection by others in the the family. *Child Development, 52*, 1274-1282.
Dance, F. E. (1967). Toward a theory of human communication. In F. E. Dance (Ed.), *Human communication theory*. New York: Holt, Rinehart & Winston.
Dantzig, A. van (1978). Het systeem van de hoop. In A. van Dantzig & A. de Swaan (red.), *Omgaan met angst in een kankerziekenhuis* (pp. 27-41). Utrecht/ Antwerpen: Aula/Spectrum. (Verboden).
Danziger, K. (1976). *Interpersonal communication*. New York: Pergamon.
Dash, J. (1980). Hypnosis for symptom amelioration. In J. Kellerman (Ed.), *Psychological aspects of childhood cancer* (pp. 215-230). Springfield, IL: Charles C Thomas.
Deasy-Spinetta, P. (1981). The school and the child with cancer. In J. J. Spinetta & P. Deasy-Spinetta (Eds.), *Living with childhood cancer* (pp. 153-168). St. Louis, MO: Mosby.
Dechert, H., & Raupach, M. (1980). *Temporal variables in speech. Studies in honour of Frieda Goldman-Eisler*. Den Haag: Mouton.
Dekking, Y. M. (1983). *S.A.S.-K Sociale Angstschaal voor Kinderen. Handleiding*. Lisse: Swets & Zeitlinger.
Dekking, Y. M., & Salentijn, M. (1979). De defensieschaal. In H. Klomp, H. Mourits, & M. Salentijn. *Sociale angst en cognitieve factoren bij kinderen*. Doctoraal werkstuk. Psychologisch Laboratorium, Vakgroep Ontwikkelingspsychologie van de Universiteit van Amsterdam.
DeLong, D. R. (1970). *Individual differences in patterns of anxiety arousal, stress-relevant information and recovery from surgery*. Unpublished doctoral dissertation, University of California, Los Angeles.
Dobkin, P. L., & Morrow, G. R. (1985). Long-term side effects in patients who have been treated succesfully for cancer. *Journal of Psychosocial Oncology, 3*(4), 23-51.
Doleys, D. M. (1977). Behavioral treatments for nocturnal enuresis in children: A review of the literature. *Psychological Bulletin, 84*, 30-54.
Dolgin, M. J., Katz, E. R., McGinty, K., & Siegel, S. E. (1985). Anticipatory nausea and vomiting in pediatric cancer patients. *Pediatrics, 75*, 547-552.
Dongen-Melman, J. E. van, Pruyn, J. F., Zanen, G. E. van, & Sanders-Woudstra, J. A. (1986). Coping with childhood cancer: A conceptual view. *Journal of Psychosocial Oncology, 4*(1/2), 147-161.
Dush, D. M., & Brodsky, M. (1981). Effects and implications of the experimental double bind. *Psychological Reports, 48*, 895-900.
Eiser, C. (1980). How leukaemia affects a child's schooling. *British Journal of Social and Clinical Psychology, 19*, 365-368.
Eiser, C. (1984). Annotation. Communicating with sick and hospitalized children. *Journal of Child Psychology and Psychiatry, 25*, 181-189.
Eiser, C., & Lansdown, R. (1977). A retrospective study of intellectual development in children treated for acute lymphoblastic leukemia. *Archives of Disease in Childhood, 52*, 525-529.
Epstein, S. (1973). Expectancy and magnitude of reaction to a noxious UCS. *Psychophysiology, 10*, 100-107.
Evans, A. E., & Edin, S. (1968). If a child must die. *New England Journal of Medicine, 278*, 138-142.
Eys, J. van, & Sullivan, M. P. (1980). Preface. In J. van Eys & M. P. Sullivan (Eds.), *Status of the curability of childhood cancers* (pp. v-vi). New York: Raven.
Ferguson, G. A. (1966). *Statistical analysis in psychology and education*. London: McGraw-Hill.
Fife, B. L. (1978). Reducing parental overprotection of the leukemic child. *Social Science and Medicine, 12*, 117-122.
Folkman, S., Schaefer, C., & Lazarus, R. S. (1979). Cognitive processes as mediators of stress and coping. In V. Hamilton & D. M. Warburton (Eds.), *Human stress and cognition: An information-processing approach*. London: Wiley.
Friedman, S. B. (1967). Care of the family of the child with cancer. *Pediatrics (Supplement), 40*, 498-504.
Friedman, S. B., Chodoff, P., Mason, J. W., & Hamburg, D. A. (1963). Behavioral observations on parents anticipating the death of a child. *Pediatrics, 32*, 610-625.

Frijda, N. H. (1986). *The Emotions*. London/Paris: Cambridge University Press/ Editions de la Maison des Sciences de l'Homme.
Frijda, N. H. (1987). *De wetten van het gevoel. Rede uitgesproken ter gelegenheid van de zevende Duijkerlezing*. Deventer: Van Loghum Slaterus.
Frijling-Schreuder, E. C. (1973). Het stervende kind. *Maandschrift voor Kindergeneeskunde, 41*, 266-271. Zie ook Discussie pp. 299-308.
Futterman, E. H., & Hoffman, I. (1973). Crisis and adaptation in the families of fatally ill children. In E. J. Anthony & C. Koupernik (Eds.), *The child and his family: The impact of disease and death* (pp. 127-143). New York: Wiley.
Gartley, W., & Bernasconi, M. (1967). The concept of death in children. *Journal of Genetic Psychology, 110*, 71-85.
George, S. L. (1980). Statistical design for pediatrics: past, present, and future. In J. van Eys & M. P. Sullivan (Eds.), *Status of the curability of childhood cancers* (pp. 47-59). New York: Raven.
Geus, G. H. de, & Last, B. F. (1983). Een bijdrage aan de validering van de BAP-schaal. *De Psycholoog, 18*, 85-89.
Gips, C. D. (1956). *How illness experiences are interpreted by hospitalized children*. Unpublished doctoral dissertation, Colombia University.
Glaser, B. G., & Strauss, A. L. (1965). *Awareness of dying*. Chicago, IL: Aldine.
Glass, D. C. (1977a). *Behaviour patterns, stress and coronary disease*. Hillsdale, NJ: Erlbaum.
Glass, D. C. (1977b). Stress, behaviour patterns, and coronary disease. *American Scientist, 65*, 177-187.
Goffman, E. (1963). *Stigma. Notes on the management of spoiled identity*. Englewood Cliffs, NJ: Prentice-Hall.
Gould, H., & Toghill, P. J. (1981). How should we talk about acute leukaemia to adult patients and their families? *British Medical Journal, 282*, 210-212.
Green, M. (1967). Care of the dying child. *Pediatrics (Supplement), 40*, 492-497.
Green, M., & Solnit, A. J. (1964). Reactions to the threatened loss of a child: A vulnerable child syndrome. Pediatric management of the dying child, Part 3. *Pediatrics, 34*, 58-66.
Greenberg, L. W., Jewett, L. S., Gluck, R. S., Champion, L. A., Leikin, S. L., Altieri, M. F., & Lipnick, R. N. (1984). Giving information for a life-threatening diagnosis. *American Journal of Diseases of Children, 138*, 649-653.
Gresnigt, H. A., & Gresnigt-Strengers, A. M. (1973). *Ouders en gezinnen met een diep zwakzinnig kind*. Lisse: Swets & Zeitlinger.
Hackett, T. P., & Weisman, A. D. (1977). Reactions to the imminence of death. In A. Monat & R. S. Lazarus (Eds.), *Stress and coping. An anthology* (pp. 324-333). New York: Colombia University Press.
Haley, J. (1976). *Problem-solving therapy*. San Francisco: Jossey-Bass.
Hansen, Y. (1973). Development of the concept of death: cognitive aspects (Doctoral dissertation, 1972). *Dissertation Abstracts International, 34*, 2b.
Harris, P. L., Olthof, T., & Meerum Terwogt, M. (1981). Children's knowledge of emotion. *Journal of Child Psychology and Psychiatry, 22*, 247-261.
Harter, S. (1979). *Children's understanding of multiple emotions: A cognitive developmental approach*. Adress presented to the ninth annual symposium of the Jean Piaget Society, May 31-June 2, Philadelphia, PA.
Heerden, J. van (1977). *Tussen psychologie en filosofie. Essays*. Meppel: Boom.
Heffron, W. A., Bommelaere, K., & Masters, R. (1973). Group discussions with the parents of leukemic children. *Pediatrics, 52*, 831-840.
Henning, J., & Fritz, G. K. (1983). School reentry in childhood cancer. *Psychosomatics, 24*, 261-269.
Heydendael, P., Tax, B., & Persoon, J. (1979). Sociological and social/ psychological variables: Definitions and measurement techniques. Chapter 8. In B. Prahl-Andersen, C. J. Kowalski, & P. H. Heydendael (Eds.), *A mixed- longitudinal, interdisciplinary study of growth and development*. New York: Academic Press.
Hilgard, J. R., & LeBaron, S. (1982). Relief of anxiety and pain in children and adolescents with cancer: Quantitative measures and clinical observations. *International Journal of Clinical and Experimental Hypnosis, 30*, 417-442.

Hofer, M. A., Wolff, C. T., Friedman, S. B., & Mason, J. W. (1972). A psychoendocrine study of bereavement. Part I. 17-Hydroxycorticosteroid excretion rates of parents following death of their children from leukemia. *Psychosomatic Medicine, 34*, 481-504.

Holmes, T. H., & Rahe, R. H. (1967). The social readjustment rating scale. *Journal of Psychosomatic Research, 11*, 213-218.

Horowitz, M. J. (1979). Psychological response to serious life events. In V. Hamilton & D. M. Warburton (Eds.), *Human stress and cognition: An information-processing approach.* London: Wiley.

Howell, D. A. (1966). A child dies. *Journal of Pediatric Surgery, 1*, 2-7.

Issner, N. (1973). Can the child be distracted from his disease? *Journal of School Health, 43*, 468-471.

Jaffe, N., O'Malley, J. E., & Koocher, G. P. (1981). Late medical consequences of childhood cancer. In G. P. Koocher & J. E. O'Malley (Eds.), *The Damocles Syndrome. Psychosocial consequences of surviving childhood cancer* (pp. 51-59). New York: McGraw-Hill.

Janis, I. L. (1969). *Stress and frustration.* New York: Harcourt Brace Jovanovich.

Janis, I. L. (1985). Coping patterns among patients with life threatening diseases. In C. D. Spielberger, I. G. Sarason, & P. B. Defares (Eds.), *Stress and anxiety, Vol. 9.* Washington, DC: Hemisphere.

Jessen, J. (1974). *Medische consumptie.* Groningen: Rijks Universiteit Groningen, Sociologisch Instituut.

Johnson, F. L., Rudolph, L. A., & Hartmann, J. R. (1979). Helping the family cope with childhood cancer. *Psychosomatics, 20*, 241-251.

Jonge, G. A. de (1969). *Kinderen met enuresis.* Academisch Proefschrift, Rijksuniversiteit te Utrecht. Assen: Van Gorcum.

Kagen-Goodheart, L. (1977). Reentry: Living with childhood cancer. *American Journal of Orthopsychiatry, 47*, 651-658.

Kalnins, I. V., Churchill, M. P., & Terry, G. E. (1980). Concurrent stresses in families with a leukemic child. *Journal of Pediatric Psychology, 5*, 81-92.

Kamphuis, R. P. (1976). *Kinderen met aangeboren hartafwijkingen en hun ouders. Een gedragswetenschappelijk onderzoek.* Academisch Proefschrift, Rijksuniversiteit te Leiden. 's Gravenhage: Pasmans.

Kaplan, D. M., Smith, A., Grobstein, R., & Fischman, S. E. (1977). Family mediation of stress. In R. H. Moos (Ed.), *Coping with physical illness* (pp. 81-96). New York: Plenum.

Karon, M. (1973). The physician and the adolescent with cancer. *Pediatric Clinics of North America, 20*, 965-973.

Karon, M., & Vernick, J. (1968). An approach to the emotional support of fatally ill children. *Clinical Pediatrics, 7*, 274-280.

Kashani, J., & Hakami, N. (1982). Depression in children and adolescents with malignancy. *Canadian Journal of Psychiatry, 27*, 474-477.

Katz, E. R., Kellerman, J., & Siegel, S. E. (1980). Behavioral distress in children with cancer undergoing medical procedures: Developmental considerations. *Journal of Consulting and Clinical Psychology, 48*, 356-365.

Kellerman, J., Rigler, D., Siegel, S. E., & Katz, E. R. (1977). Disease- related communication and depression in pediatric cancer patients. *Journal of Pediatric Psychology, 2*, 52-53.

Kellerman, J., Zeltzer, L., Ellenberg, L., Dash, J., & Rigler, D. (1980). Psychological effects of illness in adolescence. I. Anxiety, self-esteem, and perception of control. *Journal of Pediatrics, 97*, 126-131.

Kellerman, J., Zeltzer, L., Ellenberg, L., & Dash, J. (1983). Adolescents with cancer. Hypnosis for the reduction of the acute pain and anxiety associated with medical procedures. *Journal of Adolescent Health Care, 4*, 85-90.

Klomp, H., Mourits, H., & Salentijn, M. (1979). *Sociale angst en cognitieve factoren bij kinderen.* Doctoraal werkstuk. Psychologisch Laboratorium, Vakgroep Ontwikkelingspsychologie van de Universiteit van Amsterdam.

Knapp, V. S., & Hansen, H. (1973). Helping parents of children with leukemia. *Social Work, 18*, 70-75.

Knudson, A. G., & Natterson, J. M. (1960). Participation of parents in the hospital care of fatally ill children. *Pediatrics, 26*, 482-490.

Koocher, G. P. (1973). Childhood, death, and cognitive development. *Developmental Psychology, 9*, 369-375.
Koocher, G. P. (1981). Survival rates and risks. In G. P. Koocher & J. E. O'Malley (Eds.), *The Damocles Syndrome. Psychosocial consequences of surviving childhood cancer* (pp. 31-38). New York: McGraw-Hill.
Koocher, G. P., & O'Malley, J. E. (Eds.). (1981). *The Damocles Syndrome. Psychosocial consequences of surviving childhood cancer.* New York: McGraw-Hill.
Kraker, J. de, & Voûte, P. A. (1973). Humane aspecten van kanker bij kinderen. *Nederlands Tijdschrift voor Geneeskunde, 117*, 945-948.
Kramer, R. F. (1984). Living with childhood cancer: Impact on the healthy siblings. *Oncology Nursing Forum, 11*(1), 44-51.
Kreuger, A., Pehrsson, G., Gyllensköld, K., & Sjölin, S. (1981). Parent reactions to childhood malignant diseases. Experience in Sweden. *American Journal of Pediatric Hematology/Oncology, 3*, 233-238.
Krulik, T. (1978). *Loneliness in school age children with chronic life threatening illness.* Unpublished doctoral dissertation, University of California.
Kübler-Ross, E. (1969). *On death and dying.* New York: Macmillan.
Kuiken, D., & Hill, K. (1985). Double-bind communications and respondents' reluctance to affirm the validity of their self-disclosures. *Perceptual and Motor Skills, 60*, 83-95.
Kuipers, F. (1974). Het contact met de ouders. In J. F. Delemarre & P. A. Voûte (red.), *Kindertumoren* (pp. 245-254). Leiden: Stafleu.
Kupst, M. J., & Schulman, J. L. (1980). Family coping with leukemia in a child: Initial reactions. In J. L. Schulman & M. J. Kupst (Eds.), *The child with cancer* (pp. 111-128). Springfield, IL: Charles C Thomas.
Kupst, M. J., Schulman, J. L., Honig, G., Maurer, H., Morgan, E., & Fochtman, D. (1982). Family coping with childhood leukemia: One year after diagnosis. *Journal of Pediatric Psychology, 7*, 157-174.
Lange, A., & Hart, O. van der (1979). *Gedragsverandering in gezinnen.* Groningen: Wolters-Noordhoff.
Lansky, S. B. (1974). Childhood leukemia. The child psychiatrist as a member of the oncology team. *Journal of the American Academy of Child Psychiatry, 13*, 499-508.
Lansky, S. B., Black, J. L., & Cairns, N. U. (1983). Childhood cancer. Medical costs. *Cancer, 52*, 762-766.
Lansky, S. B., Cairns, G. F., Cairns, N. U., Stephenson, L., Lansky, L. L., & Garin, G. (1984). Central nervous system prophylaxis. Studies showing impairment in verbal skills and academic achievement. *American Journal of Pediatric Hematology/Oncology, 6*, 183-190.
Lansky, S. B., Cairns, N. U., Clark, G. M., Lowman, J. T., Miller, L., & Trueworthy, R. (1979). Childhood cancer: Non-medical costs of the illness. *Cancer, 42*, 403-408.
Lansky, S. B., Cairns, N. U., Hassanein, R., Wehr, J., & Lowman, J. T. (1978). Childhood cancer: Parental discord and divorce. *Pediatrics, 62*, 184-188.
Lansky, S. B., & Gendel, M. (1978). Symbiotic regressive behavior patterns in childhood malignancy. *Clinical Pediatrics, 17*, 133-138.
Lansky, S. B., Lowman, J. T., Vats, T., & Gyulay, J. (1975). School phobia in children with malignant neoplasms. *American Journal of Diseases of Children, 129*, 42-46.
Lascari, A. D., & Stehbens, J. A. (1973). The reactions of families to childhood leukemia. *Clinical Pediatrics, 12*, 210-214.
Last, B. F. (1985). De arts-ouder-kind relatie en de medische besluitvorming. In B. F. Last & P. A. Voûte (red.), *Zorgen voor kinderen met kanker* (pp. 11-18). Deventer: Van Loghum Slaterus.
Last, B. F., Veldhuizen, A. M. van, Koopman, H., & Roelofsen, J. F. (1982b). Thuiszorg bij het kind met kanker. *Maatschappelijke Gezondheidszorg, 10*(10), 8-12.
Last, B. F., Veldhuizen, A. M. van, & Ouweleen, E. (1979). *De jonge adolescent met een maligne aandoening. Een exploratief onderzoek bij dertig gezinnen.* Intern rapport. Kinderoncologisch Centrum te Amsterdam.
Last, B. F., Veldhuizen, A. M. van, & Ridder-Sluiter, J. G. de (1982a). Intelligentie en concentratievermogen van kinderen met leukemie en hun aanpassing op school. *Tijdschrift voor Kindergeneeskunde, 50*, 76-82.

Lazarus, R. S. (1966). *Psychological stress and the coping process.* New York: McGraw-Hill.
Lazarus, R. S. (1981). The costs and benefits of denial. In J. J. Spinetta & P. Deasy-Spinetta (Eds.), *Living with childhood cancer* (pp. 50-67). St. Louis, MO: Mosby.
Lazarus, R. S. (1983). The costs and benefits of denial. In S. Breznitz (Ed.), *The denial of stress* (pp. 1-30). New York: International Universities Press.
Lazarus, R. S., & Folkman, S. (1984). *Stress, appraisal and coping.* New York: Springer.
Lazarus, R. S., Kanner, A. D., & Folkman, S. (1980). Emotions: A cognitive-phenomenological analysis. In R. Plutchik & H. Kellerman (Eds.), *Theories of emotions: Vol. 1. Emotion: Theory, Research and Experience.* New York: Academic Press.
Lazarus, R. S., & Launier, R. (1978). Stress-related transactions between person and environment. In L. A. Pervin & M. Lewis (Eds.), *Perspectives in interactional psychology.* New York: Plenum.
Leeuw, E. D. de (1986). *Normering van de Amsterdamse versie van de Parental Attitude Research Instrument (A-PARI).* Universiteit van Amsterdam, Subfaculteit Opvoedkunde.
Levenson, P. M., Pfefferbaum, B. J., Copeland, D. R., & Silverberg, Y. (1982). Information preferences of cancer patients ages 11-20 years. *Journal of Adolescent Health Care, 3,* 9-13.
Ley, P. (1977). Psychological studies of doctor-patient communciation. In S. Rachman (Ed.), *Contributions to medical psychology* (Vol. 1). Oxford: Pergamon.
Li, F. P. (1977). Follow-up of survivors of childhood cancer. *Cancer (Supplement), 39,* 1776-1778.
Li, F. P., Myers, M. H., Heise, H. W., & Jaffe, N. (1978). The course of five-year survivors of cancer in childhood. *Journal of Pediatrics, 93,* 185-187.
Lindemann, E. (1944). Symptomatology and management of acute grief. *American Journal of Psychiatry, 101,* 141-148.
Longhofer, J. (1980). Dying or living?: The double bind. *Culture, Medicine and Psychiatry, 4,* 119-136.
Lowenberg, J. S. (1970). The coping behaviors of fatally ill adolescents and their parents. *Nursing Forum, 9,* 269-287.
Magni, G., Messina, C., DeLeo, D., Mosconi, A., & Carli, M. (1983). Psychological distress in parents of children with acute lymphatic leukemia. *Acta Psychiatrica Scandinavica, 68,* 297-300.
Maguire, G. P. (1983). The psychological sequelae of childhood leukemia. In W. Duncan (Ed.), *Pediatric Oncology. Recent results in cancer research* (pp. 47-57). Berlin: Springer.
Mandler, G. (1975). *Mind and emotion.* New York: Wiley.
Márky, I. (1982). Children with malignant disorders and their families. A study of the implication of the disease and its treatment on everyday life. *Acta Paediatrica Scandinavica* (Supplement 303), 1-82.
Mattson, A. (1972). Long-term physical illness in childhood: A challenge to psychosocial adaptation. *Pediatrics, 50,* 801-811.
McClelland, D. C., Atkinson, J. W., Clark, R. A., & Lowell, E. L. (1958). A scoring manual for the achievement motive. In J. W. Atkinson (Ed.), *Motives in fantasy, action and society: A method of assessment and study.* Princeton, NJ: Van Nostrand.
McIntosh, J. (1974). Processes of communication, information seeking and control associated with cancer: A selective review of the literature. *Social Science and Medicine, 8,* 167-187.
McIntosh, J. (1976). Patient's awareness and desire for information about diagnosed but undisclosed malignant disease. *Lancet, aug. 7,* 300-303.
Meadows, A. T., Massari, D. J., Fergusson, J., Gordon, J., Littman, P., & Moss, K. (1981). Declines in IQ scores and cognitive dysfunctions in children with acute lymphocytic leukaemia treated with cranial irradiation. *Lancet, nov. 7,* 1015-1018.
Mehrabian, A., & Wiener, M. (1967). Decoding of inconsistent communications. *Journal of Personality and Social Psychology, 6,* 109-114.
Messer, A. P. (1979). *Zeer moeilijk eten en moeilijk beïnvloedbaar bedplassen. Onderzoek en behandeling van een tweetal problemen uit de pediatrische psychologie.* Academisch Proefschrift, Rijksuniversiteit te Leiden.
Michael, B., & Copeland, D. (1985). Prevalence and correlates of anticipatory nausea and

vomiting in children reveiving chemotherapy. *Proceedings American Society of Clinical Oncology, 4,* 247.

Miller, S. M. (1980). When is a little information a dangerous thing? Coping with stressful events by monitoring versus blunting. In S. Levine & H. Ursin (Eds.), *Coping and Health.* New York: Plenum.

Morrow, G. R., Carpenter, P. J., & Hoagland, A. C. (1984). The role of social support in parental adjustment to pediatric cancer. *Journal of Pediatric Psychology, 9,* 317-329.

Moss, H. A., Nannis, E. D., & Poplack, D. G. (1981). The effects of prophylactic treatment of the central nervous system on the intellectual functioning of children with acute lymphocytic leukemia. *American Journal of Medicine, 71,* 47-52.

Mulhern, R. K., Crisco, J. J., & Camitta, B. M. (1981). Patterns of cummunication among pediatric patients with leukemia, parents, and physicians: Prognostic disagreements and misunderstandings. *Journal of Pediatrics, 99,* 480-483.

Murray, D. C. (1971). Talk, silence and anxiety. *Psychological Bulletin, 75,* 244-260.

Murstein, B. I. (1960). The effect of long-term illness of children on the emotional adjustment of parents. *Child Development, 31,* 157-171.

Myers, B. A. (1983). The informing interview. Enabling parents to 'hear' and cope with bad news. *American Journal of Diseases of Children, 137,* 572-577.

Nagy, M. (1948). The child's theories concerning death. *Journal of Genetic Psychology, 73,* 3-27.

Nannis, E. D., Susman, E. J., Strope, B. E., Woodruff, P. J., Hersch, S. P., Levine, A. S., & Pizzo, P. A. (1982). Correlates of control in pediatric cancer patients and their families. *Journal of Pediatric Psychology, 7,* 75-84.

Natterson, J. M., & Knudson, A. G. (1960). Observations concerning fear of death in fatally ill children and their mothers. *Psychosomatic Medicine, 22,* 456-465.

Neidhardt, M. K., & Hertl, M. (1978). Die seelische Betreuung des onkologisch kranken Kindes und seiner Eltern. *Monatsschrift für Kinderheilkunde, 126,* 479-486.

Nilsen, T. R. (1970). On defining communication. In K. Sereno & C. Mortensen (Eds.), *Foundations of communication theory.* New York: Harper & Row.

Nitschke, R., Humphrey, G. B., Sexauer, C. L., Catron, B., Wunder, S., & Jay, S. (1982). Therapeutic choices made by patients with end-stage cancer. *Journal of Pediatrics, 101,* 471-476.

Nitschke, R., Olson, R., Kaufman, K., & Funk, M. (1986). Medical staff's communication skills with family members of children with cancer. *Proceedings American Society of Clinical Oncology, 5,* 243.

Novack, D. H., Plumer, R., Smith, R. L., Ochitill, H., Morrow, G. R., & Bennett, J. M. (1979). Changes in physicians' attitudes toward telling the cancer patient. *Journal of the American Medical Association, 241,* 897-900.

Oken, D. (1961). What to tell cancer patients. *Journal of the American Medical Association, 175,* 1120-1128.

Ormel, J. (1980a). Over neuroticisme gemeten met de vragenlijst: een persoonlijkheidskenmerk of een maat voor psychosociale belasting? *Nederlands Tijdschrift voor de Psychologie, 35,* 223-241.

Ormel, J. (1980b). *Moeite met leven of een moeilijk leven. Een vervolgonderzoek naar de invloed van psychosociale belasting op het welbevinden van driehonderd Nederlanders.* Academisch Proefschrift, Rijksuniversiteit te Groningen. Groningen: Konstapel.

Osgood, C. E., Suci, G. J., & Tannenbaum, P. H. (1957). *The measurement of meaning.* Urbana, IL: University Press.

Out, J. J., & Zegveld, P. (1977). Motivatie voor ouderschap: een onderzoek. In R. Veenhoven & E. van de Wolk (red.), *Kiezen voor kinderen* (pp. 26-48). Assen: Van Gorcum.

Parker, G., & Lipscombe, P. (1979). Parental overprotection and asthma. *Journal of Psychosomatic Research, 23,* 295-299.

Parkes, C. M. (1972). *Bereavement: Studies of grief in adult life.* New York: International University Press.

Penman, R. A. (1980). *Communication processes and relationships.* London: Academic Press.

Peters, B. M. (1978). School-aged children's beliefs about causality of illness: A review of the literature. *Maternal Child Nursing, 7,* 143-155.

Pfefferbaum, B., & Levenson, P. M. (1982). Adolescent cancer patient and physician responses to a questionnaire on patient concerns. *American Journal of Psychiatry, 139,* 348-351.
Piaget, J., & Inhelder, B. (1969). *The psychology of the child.* New York: Basic Books.
Pichler, E., Richter, R., & Jürgenssen, O. A. (1982). Eltern Leukämie- und tumorkranker Kinder äussern sich zur Mitteilung der Diagnose. *Klinische Pädiatrie, 194,* 94-99.
Pinkel, D. (1980). Criteria for biological cure of cancer. In J. van Eys & M. P. Sullivan (Eds.), *Status of the curability of childhood cancers* (pp. 21-25). New York: Raven.
Plank, E. (1964). Death on a children's ward. *Medical Times, 92,* 638-644.
Ploeg, H. M. van der (1981). *Zelf-Beoordelings Vragenlijst. Handleiding, Addendum.* Lisse: Swets & Zeitlinger.
Ploeg, H. M. van der, Defares, P. B., & Spielberger, C. D. (1980). *Handleiding bij de Zelf-Beoordelings Vragenlijst ZBV. Een nederlandstalige bewerking van de Spielberger State-Trait Anxiety Inventory, Stai-DY.* Lisse: Swets & Zeitlinger.
Powazek, M., Schijving, J., Goff, J. R., Paulson, M. A., & Stagner, S. (1980). Psychosocial ramifications of childhood leukemia: One year post- diagnosis. In J. L. Schulman & M. J. Kupst (Eds.), *The child with cancer* (pp. 143-145). Springfield, IL: Charles C Thomas.
Quinton, D., & Rutter, M. (1976). Early hospital admissions and later disturbances of behaviour: An attempted replication of Douglas' findings. *Developmental Medicine and Child Neurology, 18,* 447-459.
Rahe, R. H. (1974). The pathway between subjects recent life changes and their near-future illness reports: representative results and methodological issues. In B. S. Dohrenwend & B. P. Dohrenwend (Eds.), *Stressful life events: their nature and effects* (pp. 73-87). New York: Wiley.
Rando, T. A. (1983). An investigation of grief and adaptation in parents whose children have died from cancer. *Journal of Pediatric Psychology, 8,* 3-20.
Reissland, N. (1985). The development of concepts of simultaneity in children's understanding of emotions. *Journal of Child Psychology and Psychiatry, 26,* 811-824.
Richardson, S., Dohrenwend, B., & Klein, D. (1965). *Interviewing. Its forms and functions.* New York: Basic Books.
Richmond, J. B., & Waisman, H. A. (1955). Psychologic aspects of management of children with malignant diseases. *American Journal of Diseases of Children, 89,* 42-47.
Romsdahl, M. M. (1980). Status of the curability of solid tumors. In J. van Eys & M. P. Sullivan (Eds.), *Status of the curability of childhood cancers* (pp. 63-67). New York: Raven.
Rothbaum, F., Weisz, J. R., & Snyder, S. S. (1982). Changing the world and changing the self: A two-process model of perceived control. *Journal of Personality and Social Psychology, 42,* 5-37.
Rowland, J. H., Glidewell, O. J., Sibley, R. F., Holland, J. C., Tull, R., Berman, A., Brecher, M. L., Harris, M., Glicksman, A. S., Forman, E., Jones, B., Cohen, M. E., Duffner, P. K., & Freeman, A. I. (1984). Effects of different forms of central nervous system prophylaxis on neuropsychologic function in childhood leukemia. *Journal of Clinical Oncology, 2,* 1327-1335.
Ruesch, J., & Bateson, G. (1951). *Communication: The social matrix of psychiatry.* New York: Norton.
Rutter, M. (1972). *Maternal deprivation reassessed.* Harmondsworth, England: Penguin.
Saarni, C. (1979). Children's understanding of display rules for expressive behavior. *Developmental Psychology, 15,* 424-429.
Sarason, S. B., Davidson, K. S., Lighthall, F. F., Waite, R. R., & Ruebush, B. K. (1960). *Anxiety in elementary school children.* New York: Wiley.
Schaefer, E. S. (1959). A circumplex model for maternal behavior. *Journal of Abnormal Social Psychology, 59,* 226.
Schaefer, E. S., & Bell, R. Q. (1958). Development of a parental attitude research instrument. *Child Development, 29,* 339-361.
Schowalter, J. E. (1970). The child's reaction to his own terminal illness. In B. Schoenberg, A. C. Carr, D. Peretz, & A. H. Kutcher (Eds.), *Loss and grief* (pp. 51-69). New York: Colombia University Press.
Schreurs, P. J., Tellegen, B., & Willige, G. van de (1986a). Coping: Theoretische aspecten

en enkele operationalisaties. In P. J. Schreurs & R. Rombouts (red.), *Omgaan met ernstige ziekten* (pp. 4-18). Lisse: Swets & Zeitlinger.

Schreurs, P. J., Willige, G. van de, Tellegen, B., & Brosschot, G. (1986b). *De Utrechtse Coping-Lijst: UCL. Handleiding.* Vakgroep Klinische Psychologie van de Rijksuniversiteit te Utrecht.

Seligman, M. E. (1975). *Helplessness.* San Francisco: Freeman.

Selye, H. (1956). *The stress of life.* New York: McGraw-Hill.

Sereno, K., & Bodaken, E. (1975). *Trans-Per understanding human communication.* Boston: Houghton Mifflin.

Share, L. (1972). Family communication in the crisis of a child's fatal illness: A literature review and analysis. *Omega, 3,* 187-201.

Siegel, S. (1956). *Nonparametric statistics for the behavioral sciences.* New York: McGraw-Hill.

Siegel, S. E. (1980). The current outlook for childhood cancer - the medical background. In J. Kellerman (Ed.), *Psychological aspects of childhood cancer* (pp. 5-13). Springfield, IL: Charles C Thomas.

Singer, J. E. (1984). Some issues in the study of coping. *Cancer (Supplement), 53,* 2303-2313.

Sinnema, G. (1984). *Chronisch zieke adolescenten. Zelfstandigheidsontwikkeling en ziektebeleving bij adolescenten met cystic fibrosis.* Academisch Proefschrift, Rijskuniversiteit te Utrecht. Utrecht: Bohn, Scheltema & Holkema.

Sjamsoedin-Visser, E. J., & Leeuwen, E. F. van (1983). Acute leukemie bij kinderen. In K. Punt & R. L. Verwilghen (red.), *Acute leukemie* (pp. 74-85). Alphen aan den Rijn: Stafleu.

Slavin, L. A., O'Malley, J. E., Koocher, G. P., & Foster, D. J. (1982). Communication of the cancer diagnosis to pediatric patients: Impact on long-term adjustment. *American Journal of Psychiatry, 139,* 179-183.

Sluzki, C. E., & Véron, E. (1971). The double bind as a universal pathogenic situation. *Family Process, 10,* 397-409.

Smith, E. K. (1976). Effect of double-bind communication on the anxiety level of normals. *Journal of Abnormal Psychology, 85,* 356-363.

Sontag, S. (1979). *Illness as a metaphor.* London: Lane.

Spielberger, C. D., Edwards, C. D., Lushene, R. E., Montuori, J., & Platzek, D. (1973). *STAIC Preliminary Manual for the State-Trait Anxiety Inventory for Children.* Palo Alto, CA: Consulting Psychologists Press.

Spielberger, C. D., Gorsuch, R. L., & Lushene, R. E. (1970). *STAI Manual for the State-Trait Anxiety Inventory.* Palo Alto, CA: Consulting Psychologists Press.

Spinetta, J. J. (1972). *Death anxiety in leukemic children.* Unpublished doctoral dissertation, University of Southern California, Los Angeles. (University Microfilms No. 72-26,056).

Spinetta, J. J. (1974). The dying child's awareness of death: A review. *Psychological Bulletin, 81,* 256-260.

Spinetta, J. J. (1978). Communication patterns in families dealing with life-threatening illness. In O. J. Sahler (Ed.), *The child and death* (pp. 43-51). St. Louis, MO: Mosby.

Spinetta, J. J. (1980). Disease-related communication: How to tell. In J. Kellerman (Ed.), *Psychological aspects of childhood cancer* (pp. 257-269). Springfield, IL: Charles C Thomas.

Spinetta, J. J., & Deasy-Spinetta, P. (1981). Talking with children who have a life-threatening illness. In J. J. Spinetta & P. Deasy-Spinetta (Eds.), *Living with childhood cancer* (pp. 234-252). St. Louis, MO: Mosby.

Spinetta, J. J., & Maloney, L. J. (1975). Death anxiety in the outpatient leukemic child. *Pediatrics, 56,* 1034-1037.

Spinetta, J. J., & Maloney, L. J. (1978). The child with cancer: patterns of communication and denial. *Journal of Consulting and Clinical Psychology, 46,* 1540-1541.

Spinetta, J. J., Rigler, D., & Karon, M. (1973). Anxiety in the dying child. *Pediatrics, 52,* 841-845.

Spinetta, J. J., Swarner, J. A., & Sheposh, J. P. (1981). Effective parental coping following the death of a child from cancer. *Journal of Pediatric Psychology, 6,* 251-263.

SPSS *Statistical package for the social sciences.* (2nd ed.). (1975). New York: McGraw-Hill.
SPSS *Update 7-9.* (1981). New York: McGraw-Hill.
STAP-Statistical Appendix User's Manual: Vol. 2. Association, Distance, Cluster. (1980). TC-Publication nr. 102. Amsterdam: Technisch Centrum FSW, University of Amsterdam.
STAP-Statistical Appendix User's Manual: Vol. 5. Item analysis. (1980). TC-Publication nr. 105. Amsterdam: Technisch Centrum FSW, University of Amsterdam.
Steensel-Moll, H. A. van (1983). *Childhood leukaemia in the Netherlands. A register based epidemiologic study.* Academisch Proefschrift, Erasmus Universiteit Rotterdam.
Stotland, E. (1969). *The psychology of hope. An integration of experimental, clinical, and social approaches.* San Francisco: Jossey-Bass.
Susman, E. J., Hersch, S. P., Nannis, E. D., Strope, B. E., Woodruff, R. J., Pizzo, P. A., & Levine, A. S. (1982). Conceptions of cancer: The perspectives of child and adolescent patients and their families. *Journal of Pediatric Psychology, 7,* 253-260.
Susman, E. J., Hollenbeck, A. R., Nannis, E. D., Strope, B. E., Hersch, S. P., Levine, A. S., & Pizzo, P. A. (1981). A prospective naturalistic study of the impact of an intensive medical treatment on the social behavior of child and adolescent cancer patients. *Journal of Applied Developmental Psychology, 2,* 29-47.
Susman, E. J., Hollenbeck, A. R., Strope, B. E., Hersch, S. P., Levine, A. S., & Pizzo, P. A. (1980). Separation-deprivation and childhood cancer: A conceptual reevaluation. In J. Kellerman (Ed.), *Psychological aspects of childhood cancer* (pp. 155-170). Springfield, IL: Charles C Thomas.
Suurmeijer, T. P. (1980). *Kinderen met epilepsie. Een onderzoek naar de invloed van een ziekte op kind en gezin.* Academisch Proefschrift, Rijksuniversiteit te Groningen.
Swaan, A. de (1982). *De mens is de mens een zorg.* Amsterdam: Meulenhoff.
Swain, H. L. (1976). The concept of death in children. (Doctoral dissertation, 1975). *Dissertation Abstracts International, 37,* 2a.
Toch, R. (1964). Management of the child with a fatal disease. *Clinical Pediatrics, 3,* 418-427.
Townes, B. D., Wold, D. A., & Holmes, T. H. (1974). Parental adjustment to childhood leukemia. *Journal of Psychosomatic Research, 18,* 9-14.
Tropauer, A., Franz, M. N., & Dilgard, V. W. (1970). Psychological aspects of the care of children with cystic fibrosis. *American Journal of Diseases of Children, 119,* 424-432.
Turk, J. (1964). Impact of cystic fibrosis on family functioning. *Pediatrics, 34,* 67-71.
Veeneklaas, G. M. (1960). Meedelen van en mee-delen in de diagnose (I). *Nederlands Tijdschrift voor Geneeskunde, 104,* 1405-1409.
Veeneklaas, G. M. (1962). Meedelen van en mee-delen in de diagnose (II). *Nederlands Tijdschrift voor Geneeskunde, 106,* 1929-1931.
Veeneklaas, G. M. (1964a). Meedelen van en mee-delen in de diagnose (III). Het sterfbed. *Nederlands Tijdschrift voor Geneeskunde, 108,* 2393-2396.
Veeneklaas, G. M. (1964b). Meedelen van en mee-delen in de diagnose (IV). De rouw. *Nederlands Tijdschrift voor Geneeskunde, 108,* 2441-2444.
Veeneklaas, G. M. (1977). Emancipatie betreffende de infauste prognose op de kinderleeftijd. *Nederlands Tijdschrift voor Geneeskunde, 121,* 305-308.
Veldhuizen, A. M. van (1985). De beleving van het kind. In B. F. Last & P. A. Voûte (red.), *Zorgen voor kinderen met kanker* (pp. 21-41). Deventer: Van Loghum Slaterus.
Vernick, J., & Karon, M. (1965). Who's afraid of death on a leukemia ward? *American Journal of Diseases of Children, 109,* 393-397.
Vernon, D. T., Foley, J. M., Sipowicz, R. R., & Schulman, J. L. (1965). *The psychological responses of children to hospitalization and illness.* Springfield, IL: Charles C Thomas.
Visser, A. Ph. (1982). Angst en informatieverstrekking bij chirurgische patiënten. In H. M. van der Ploeg & P. B. Defares (red.), *Stress en angst in de medische situatie.* Alphen aan den Rijn: Stafleu.
Voûte, P. A. (1985). Kanker op de kinderleeftijd: de ziekte en de behandelingsmogelijkheden. In B. F. Last & P. A. Voûte (red.), *Zorgen voor kinderen met kanker* (pp. 133-145). Deventer: Van Loghum Slaterus.
Voûte, P. A., Vos, A., Delemarre, J. F., Kraker, J. de, Burgers, J. M., & Dobbenburgh, O. A. van (1980). The persistent challenge of neuroblastoma. In J. van Eys & M. P. Sullivan (Eds.), *Status of the curability of childhood cancers* (pp. 145-161). New York: Raven.

Waal, F. C. de (1973). Het kind dat sterven gaat. *Maandschrift voor Kindergeneeskunde, 41,* 260-265. Zie ook Discussie pp. 299-308.
Waard, F. de (1983). Epidemiologie van de leukemieën. In K. Punt & R. L. Verwilghen (red.), *Acute leukemie* (pp. 13-26). Alphen aan den Rijn: Stafleu.
Waechter,E. H. (1971). Children's awareness of fatal illness. *American Journal of Nursing, 71,* 1168-1172.
Watzlawick, P., Beavin, J. H., & Jackson, D. D. (1967). *Pragmatics of human communications.* New York: Norton.
Weisman, A. D. (1972). *On dying and denying. A psychiatric study of terminality.* New York: Behavioral Publications.
Weisman, A. D. (1974). Is mourning necessary? In B. Schoenberg, A. C. Carr, A. H. Kutcher, D. Peretz, & I. Goldberg (Eds.), *Anticipatory Grief* (pp. 171-181). New York: Columbia University Press.
White, R. W. (1974). Strategies of adaptation: An attempt at systematic description. In G. V. Coelho, D. A. Hamburg, & J. E. Adams (Eds.), *Coping and adaptation.* New York: Basic Books.
White, E., Elsom, B., & Prawat, R. (1978). Children's conceptions of death. *Child Development, 49,* 307-310.
Wiener, M., Devoe, S., Rubinow, S., & Geller, J. (1972). Nonverbal behavior and nonverbal communication. *Psychological Review, 79,* 185-214.
Wiggers, M. (1984). *Emotion recognition in children and adults.* Academisch Proefschrift, Katholieke Universiteit te Nijmegen.
Wilde, G. J. (1970). *Neurotische labiliteit gemeten volgens de vragenlijstmethode. Tweede vermeerderde uitgave.* Amsterdam: Van Rossum.
Wit, C. A. de (1985). *Depressie bij kinderen. Psychologische theorie en operationalisering.* Academisch Proefschrift, Universiteit van Amsterdam. Leuven: Acco.
Wolff, C. T., Friedman, S. B., Hofer, M. A., & Mason, J. W. (1964). Relationship between psychological defenses and mean urinary 17-hydroxycorticosteroid excretion rates. A predictive study of parents of fatally ill children (Parts 1 and 2). *Psychosomatic Medicine, 26,* 576-609.
Wolters, W. H. (1970). Het stervende kind in het ziekenhuis. *Maandschrift voor Kindergeneeskunde, 38,* 131-141.
Wijmans-Bruggeman, W. (1981). *De beleving van het kind met kanker en de kommunikatiewijze van de ouders over de ziekte.* Scriptie Orthopedagogiek M.O.-A. Stichting Nutsseminarium aan de Universiteit van Amsterdam.
Zeeuw, J. de (1976). *Algemene Psychodiagnostiek I. Testmethoden.* Amsterdam: Swets & Zeitlinger.
Zeltzer, L., Kellerman, J., Ellenberg, L., Dash, J., & Rigler, D. (1980). Psychologic effects of illness in adolescence. II. Impact of illness in adolescents -crucial issues and coping styles. *Journal of Pediatrics, 97,* 132-138.
Zeltzer, L., Kellerman, J., Ellenberg, L., & Dash, J. (1983). Hypnosis for reduction of vomiting associated with chemotherapy and disease in adolescents with cancer. *Journal of Adolescent Health Care, 4,* 77-84.
Zeltzer, L., & LeBaron, S. (1982). Hypnosis and nonhypnotic techniques for reduction of pain and anxiety during painful procedures in children and adolescents with cancer. *Journal of Pediatrics, 101,* 1032-1035.

11. Appendices

Appendix I
Biographical and disease characteristics of the sample

I.1 Composition of the sample

	n	%	Girls n	Girls %	Boys n	Boys %
Children with cancer:						
Total group	82	100.0	39	47.6	43	52.4
4 to 7 year olds	26	31.7	13	50.0	13	50.0
8 to 12 year olds	32	39.0	14	43.8	18	56.3
13 to 16 year olds	24	29.3	12	50.0	12	50.0
Parents:						
Total group	159	100.0				
Mothers	81	50.9				
Fathers	78	49.1				
Two-parent family	77	93.9				
Single parent family	5	6.1				

I.2 Age of the children and the parents

	mean (years)	SD (years)	range (years;months)
Children with cancer:			
Total group	10.24	3.52	4;0-16;11
4 to 7 year olds	5.65	1.09	4;0-7;11
8 to 12 year olds	9.94	1.24	8;1-12;3
13 to 16 year olds	14.08	1.14	13;0-16;11
Parents:			
Total group	38.11	5.50	25-54
Mothers	36.96	5.69	25-52
Fathers	39.29	5.07	28-54

I.3 Educational level of the parents

	total group %	mothers %	fathers %
Completed education:	(n=159)	(n=81)	(n=78)
Primary school, Secondary school, occupational and vocational training	49.6	62.9	35.8
Extra occupational and vocational training	25.1	18.5	32.0
Pre-university education	8.1	7.4	8.9
College	6.9	3.7	10.2
Higher education (University)	10.0	7.4	12.8

I.4 Socio-economic status of the family (n=82) (based on education and job/profession)

	%
High	20.7
Middle	29.2
Low	50.0

I.5 Size of family (n=82)

	%
Number of children:	
One child	9.7
Two children	52.4
Three children	24.3
Four children	10.9
Five children	1.2
Six children	1.2

I.6 Age of the children (including the sick child) (n=201)

	%
0-1 years	1.4
1-4 years	5.9
4-6 years	10.4
6-12 years	41.7
12-21 years	37.8
>21 years	2.4

I.7 Birth rank of the sick child (n=82)

	%
Only child	9.7
Oldest child	29.2
Middle child	14.6
Youngest child	46.3

I.8 Nature of the children's diagnosis (n=82)

Nature of the diagnosis	%
Acute lymphocytic leukemia	22
Acute myeloid leukemia	1
Morbus Hodgkin	17
Osteosarcoma	10
Wilms' tumor	9
Lymphosarcoma	9
Rhabdomyosarcoma	9
Burkitt's lymphoma	4
Ewing's sarcoma	4
Malignant hystiocytosis	4
Medulloblastoma	2
Neuroblastoma	2
Fibrosarcoma	1
Endodermal sinus tumor	1
Malignant teratoma	1
Nasopharynx carcinoma	1
Thyroid gland carcinoma	1
Undifferentiated sarcoma	1

I.9 Status of disease and treatment for the children (n=82)

	%
Good prognosis	60
Poor prognosis	40
(Former) relapse or recurrence	12
In continuous first remission	82
In (subsequent) remission	88
Undergoing treatment	39
Treatment finished	61

I.10 Treatment duration, number of hospital admissions, and number of days in hospital for the children (n=82)

	mean	range
Treatment duration in months	11	3-26
Number of hospital admissions	8	1-31
Number of days in hospital	72	12-168

Appendix II
Intercorrelations between the communication variables and emotion variables of the children and the parents

II.1 Intercorrelations between the communication variables (CSP) of the parents (n=159)

	ID	IP	CE	EW	EG	CIC	CIP	IC
ID	1.00	.43**	.17*	.26**	.11	.06	.05	.21**
IP			.03	.11	.17*	.01	.12	.20*
CE				.09	.22**	.13	-.01	-.10
EW					.18*	.17*	.04	.01
EG						.20*	.09	.12
CIC							.27**	.01
CIP								.12
IC								1.00

* = p<.05
** = p<.01
For the abbreviatons used, see Outline of instruments, section 5.3.

II.2 Intercorrelations between the anxiety variables of the child

	ST-AT	ST-AS	LAT-HP	LAT-ITW	BLOCK-HP	BLOCK-ITW	HP-FP	HP-DA	IBC-AF
ST-AT	1.00	.44**	.12	.14	-.30	.05	-.31	.44*	.24
ST-AS			.28	.21	.05	.03	-.14	.15	.19
LAT-HP				.74**	.05	-.07	-.02	.06	—
LAT-ITW					-.20	.10	.03	.08	.13
BLOCK-HP						.44*	-.05	.18	—
BLOCK-ITW							.05	.14	-.14
HP-FP								-.16	—
HP-DA									—
IBC-AF									1.00

* = p<.05
** = p<.01
For the abbreviations used, see Outline of instruments, section 5.3.

II.3 Intercorrelations between the depression variables of the child

	DQC	NE-se	NE-ese	NE-f	HP-LI	HP-F	HP-G	IBC-LI	IBC-P
DQC	1.00	.87**	.34*	.65**	.06	.34	.24	.25	.17
NE-se			.37**	.46**	.15	.32	.12	-.05	.29
NE-ese				.24	-.12	-.13	-.12	.23	.25
NE-f					-.10	.05	.08	.12	.23
HP-LI						.15	.31*	–	–
HP-F							.30*	–	–
HP-G								–	–
IBC-LI									.13
IBC-P									1.00

* = p<.05
** = p<.01

For the abbreviations used, see Outline of instruments, section 5.3.

II.4 Intercorrelations between the emotion variables of the parents (n=159)

	W-P	W-PS	SRQ-AS	MC-S	MC-D	PI	IBP-LI	IBP-AI	IBP-P	IBP-H	IBP-AK	IBP-G
W-P	1.00	.58**	.42**	.17*	.27**	.19*	.35**	.34**	.12	.20*	.35**	.14
W-PS			.37**	.24**	.38**	.11	.26**	.18*	.05	.13	.28**	.08
SRQ-AS				.14	.20*	.25**	.19*	.23**	.02	.05	.17*	.12
MC-S					.27**	-.09	-.07	-.02	-.01	-.08	.03	-.01
MC-D						-.05	.14	.09	-.05	.01	.18*	.05
PI							.08	.29**	.10	.17	-.01	.06
IBP-LI								.51**	.18*	.35**	.55**	.49**
IBP-AI									.27**	.53**	.43**	.44**
IBP-P										.24**	.12	.15
IBP-H											.30**	.39**
IBP-AK												.43**
IBP-G												1.00

* = p<.05
** = p<.01

For the abbreviations used, see Outline of instruments, section 5.3.

II.5 Intercorrelations between the behavioral assessment scales (BAP) for the parents (n=159)

	CR	ChD	OI	NA
CR	1.00	.38**	.00	.40**
ChD			.53**	.51**
OI				.29**
NA				1.00

** = p<.01 For the abbreviations used, see Outline of instruments, section 5.3.

II.6 Intercorrelations between the problem behavior assessment scales (PBAP) for the parents (n=159)

	SL	B	E	SC
SL	1.00	.14	.24**	.33**
B			.06	.05
E				.28**
SC				1.00

** = p<.01
For the abbreviations used, see Outline of instruments, section 5.3.

Appendix III
Correlations between the communication variables and emotion variables, on the one hand, and the information scales and defense scale, on the other hand

III.1 Pearson correlations (r) between the communication variables (CSP) of the parents, on the one hand, and the information scales (IQC) and the defense scale (DESC) for the children (8 to 16 years), on the other hand (n=56)

Communication variables of the parents	Information scales			Defense scale
	sources r	obstacles r	needs r	r
Information about the diagnosis	.29*	-.01	.12	-.07
Information about the prognosis	.21	.04	-.06	-.16
Communication about the child's emotional experience	.10	-.01	.13	-.29*
Expression of worries	-.05	.02	.06	-.01
Expression of grief	-.19	.10	.27*	-.02
Communication about the disease at the child's initiative	-.09	.11	.22	-.16
Communication about the disease at the parents' initiative	.23	-.20	.07	.15
Indirect communication	-.06	.12	.33*	-.25

* = $p<.05$

III.2 Pearson correlations r >.20 between the emotion variables, on the one hand, and the information scales (IQC) and the defense scale (DESC) for the children (8-16 years), on the other hand

Emotion variables	n	Information scales sources r	Information scales obstacles r	Information scales needs r	Defense scale r
Anxiety variables:					
Anxiety trait (ST-AT)	56	-.43**	.42**		-.59**
Anxiety-state (ST-AS)	56	-.25	.30*		-.22
Anxiety assessment by the mother (BAP-NA)	55		.25		
Latency (HP)	32		-.23		
Latency (ITW)	56				-.28*
Blocks (HP)	32	-.24			.49**
Blocks (ITW)	56	-.32	.25		
Diffuse anxiety (HP-DA)	32	-.24		-.25	-.43*
Anxiety and frustration (IBC-AF)	24				-.37
Depression variables:					
Depression (DQC)	56	-.45**	.33*		-.52**
Negative self-esteem (NE-se)	56	-.48**	.29*		-.41**
Negative expectations for the future (NE-f)	56				-.38*
Depression assessment by the mother (BAP-ChD)	56				-.27*
Depression assessment by the father (BAP-ChD)	56				-.29*
Frustration (HP-F)	32	-.24			
Pessimism (IBC-P)	24	-.33	.24		-.47*

* = p<.05
** = p<.01

III.3 *Pearson correlations r >.20 between the variables experience of family relations (FRT) and the variables behavioral problems (BAP and PBAP), on the one hand, and the information scales (IQC) and defense scale (DESC) for the children (8 to 16 years), on the other hand*

Emotion variables	n	Information scales			Defense scale
		sources r	obstacles r	needs r	r
Experience of family relations:					
Positive feelings towards the mother (FRT-PM)	56				-.28*
Negative feelings towards the father (FRT-NF)	54	-.23			
Negative feelings towards siblings (FRT-NS)	50				-.35*
Behavioral problems:					
Calm vs. rebellious behavior assessed by the mother (BAP-CR)	55	-.24	.21		
Calm vs. rebellious behavior assessed by the father (BAP-CR)	52		.29*		
Sleeping problems assessed by the mother (PBAP-SL)	55		.38**		-.22
Bed-wetting assessed by the mother (PBAP-B)	55	-.30*	.31		
Bed-wetting assessed by the father (PBAP-B)	52	-.21			

* = p<.05
** = p<.01

Appendix IV
Correlations between the information-seeking behavior scale and the communication variables, emotion variables, and the coping scale

IV.1 Pearson correlations r >.20 between the information-seeking behavior scale (ISP) and the communication variables (CSP) of the mothers (n=81) and fathers (n=78)

Communication variables	Information-seeking behavior scale	
	mothers r	fathers r
Information about the diagnosis	.25*	.38**
Information about the prognosis	.21	.28*
Communication about the emotional experience		.22
Expression of worries		.28*
Communication about the disease at the father's initiative		.35*
Indirect communication	-.22	

* = p<.05
** = p<.01

IV.2 Pearson correlations r >.20 between the information-seeking behavior scale (ISP) and the emotion variables of the fathers (n=78)

Emotion variables	Information-seeking behavior scale fathers r
Direct measures:	
Pessimism about the course of the child's illness (PC)	.27*
Projective measures:	
Anxiety and insecurity (IBP-AI)	.37**
Helplessness (IBP-H)	.22

* = p<.05
** = p<.01

IV.3 *Pearson correlations r >.20 between the information-seeking behavior scale (ISP) and the coping scale (UCL) for the mothers (n=81) and fathers (n=78)*

	Information-seeking behavior scale	
	mothers	fathers
Coping scale	r	r
Active problem-solving		.33**
Palliative reactions		.28*
Avoidance and wait-and-see attitude	-.26*	
Seeking social support		.29*
Depressive reaction pattern		
Expression of emotions/anger		.37**
Comforting cognitions		.26*

* = p<.05
** = p<.01

Appendix V
Means and standard deviations of the communication variables and emotion variables of the children and the parents

V.1 Means and standard deviations of the communication variables of the parents

Communication variables	One or both parents (n=82) mean	SD	Mothers (n=81) mean	SD	Fathers (n=78) mean	SD	Scale range
Information about the diagnosis	7.20	2.31	6.14	2.58	5.71	2.99	0-10
Information about the prognosis	2.39	1.70	1.67	1.70	1.83	1.84	0-4
Communication about the child's emotional experience	1.28	.77	1.13	.74	1.08	.79	0-2
Expression of worries	.67	.48	.62	.50	.53	.50	0-1
Expression of grief	.73	.45	.72	.45	.37	.49	0-1
Communication about the disase at the child's initiative	1.37	1.09	1.07	1.06	.77	.98	0-3
Communication about the disease at the parent's initiative	.99	1.13	.64	1.00	.63	1.01	0-3
Indirect communication	.71	.46	.62	.49	.61	.45	0-1

V.2 Means and standard deviations of the anxiety variables of the total group of children

Anxiety variables	n	mean	SD	Scale range
Direct measures:				
Anxiety trait (ST-AT) (8 to 16 year olds)	56	35.55	5.72	20-60
Anxiety-state (ST-AS) (8 to 16 year olds)	56	31.02	4.82	20-60
Indirect measures:				
Latency (HP) (4 to 12 year olds)	58	16.18	15.68	( )
Latency (ITW) (8 to 16 year olds)	56	4.88	6.45	( )
Blocks (HP) (4 to 12 year olds)	58	3.79	7.20	( )
Blocks (ITW) (8 to 16 year olds)	56	1.21	2.21	( )
Projective measures:				
Fear of pain and procedures (HP-FP) (4 to 12 year olds)	58	12.42	8.39	( )
Diffuse anxiety (HP-DA) (4 to 12 year olds)	58	5.04	5.78	( )
Anxiety and frustration (IBC-AF) (13 to 16 year olds)	24	28.58	6.51	12-48

( ) = unlimited scale range

V.3 *Means and standard deviations of the anxiety variables of the children by age group*

Anxiety variables	4 to 7 year olds (n=26)		8 to 12 year olds (n=32)		13 to 16 year olds (n=24)	
	mean	SD	mean	SD	mean	SD
Direct measures:						
Anxiety trait (ST-AT)	—	—	37.63	6.27	32.79	6.25
Anxiety-state (ST-AS)	—	—	31.41	4.95	30.50	5.08
Indirect measures:						
Latency (HP)	18.35	15.66	14.35	15.72	—	—
Latency (ITW)	—	—	4.63	6.28	5.21	6.78
Blocks (HP)	6.58	9.66	1.45	2.57	-	-
Blocks (ITW)	—	—	1.53	2.58	.79	1.53
Projective measures:						
Fear of pain and procedures (HP-FP)	15.23	10.29	10.06	5.53	—	—
Diffuse anxiety (HP-DA)	6.96	7.82	3.42	2.38	—	—
Anxiety and frustration (IBC-AF)	—	—	—	—	28.58	6.51

V.4 *Means and standard deviations of the depression variables and positive feelings of the total group of children*

Depression variables/Positive feelings	n	mean	SD	Scale range
Direct measures:				
Depression (DQC) (8 to 16 year olds)	56	25.38	16.32	0-92
Negative self-esteem (NE-se) (8 to16 year olds)	56	3.73	3.02	0-15
Negative evaluation of social environment (NE-ese) (8 to 16 year olds)	56	2.71	11.02	0-7
Negative expectations for the future (NE-f) (8 to 16 year olds)	56	2.20	2.00	0-8
Projective measures:				
Loneliness and isolation (HP-LI) (4 to 12 year olds)	58	33.32	17.60	( )
Frustration (HP-F) (4 to 12 year olds)	58	20.82	7.73	( )
Grief (HP-G) (4 to 12 year olds)	58	8.16	4.20	( )
Loneliness and isolation (IBC-LI) (13 to 16 year olds)	24	5.75	2.15	3-12
Pessimism (IBC-P) (13 to 16 year olds)	24	4.08	1.50	2-8
Positive feelings (HP-P) (4 to 12 year olds)	58	22.86	10.63	( )

( ) = unlimited scale range

V.5 Means and standard deviations of the depression variables and positive feelings of the children by age group

Depression variables/ Positive feelings	4 to 7 year olds (n=26)		8 to 12 year olds (n=32)		13 to 16 year olds (n=24)	
	mean	SD	mean	SD	mean	SD
Direct measures:						
Depression (DQC)	–	–	29.47	17.28	19.92	13.42
Negative self-esteem (NE-se)	–	–	4.56	3.26	2.63	2.28
Negative evaluation of social environment (NE-ese)	–	–	4.16	14.46	.79	1.18
Negative expectations for the future (NE-f)	–	–	2.13	1.90	2.29	2.18
Projective measures:						
Loneliness and isolation (HP-LI)	42.31	19.83	25.77	11.04	–	–
Frustration (HP-F)	23.50	6.69	18.58	7.94	–	–
Grief (HP-G)	9.38	5.35	7.13	2.58	–	–
Loneliness and isolation (IBC-LI)	–	–	–	–	5.75	2.15
Pessimism (IBC-P)	–	–	–	–	4.08	1.50
Positive feelings (HP-P)	25.00	11.52	21.06	9.65	–	–

V.6 Means and standard deviations of the Family Relations Test (FRT) for the 4 to 7 year old children (n=26) and the 8 to 16 year old children (n=56)

Family Relations Test	mean	SD
4 to 7 year olds		
Positive feelings towards:		
mother	5.04	3.18
father	4.27	2.92
siblings	4.72	2.24
Negative feelings towards:		
mother	1.37	2.11
father	4.13	4.42
siblings	4.61	4.12
8 to 16 year olds		
Positive feelings towards:		
mother	10.50	5.14
father	7.04	4.26
siblings	8.09	5.38
Negative feelings towards:		
mother	2.42	2.01
father	5.32	5.06
siblings	13.16	7.21

V.7 Means and standard deviations of the subscales of the behavioral assessment scale (BAP) and the problem behavior assessment scale (PBAP) for the group of mothers (n=81) and the group of fathers (n=78)

Behavioral problems	mothers mean	SD	fathers mean	SD	scale range
BAP subscales:					
Calm versus rebellious behavior (BAP-CR)	40.20	12.15	43.09	11.37	11-77
Cheerful versus depressed behavior (BAP-ChD)	19.81	7.89	20.71	7.39	8-56
Open versus introvert behavior (BAP-OI)	13.54	6.15	13.38	5.77	5-35
Not anxious versus anxious behavior (BAP-NA)	10.28	3.82	9.79	3.57	3-21
PBAP subscales:					
Sleeping problems (PBAP-SL)	1.40	1.54	1.24	1.41	0-5
Bed-wetting (PBAP-B)	.30	.70	.22	.60	0-2
Eating problems (PBAP-E)	.86	1.16	.99	1.16	0-3
Problems at school (PBAP-SC)	.29	.61	.25	.63	0-3

V.8 *Means and standard deviations of the emotion variables of the mothers (n=81) and the fathers (n=78).*

Emotion variables	mothers mean	SD	fathers mean	SD	scale range
Direct measures:					
Psychological stress reactions (W-P)	18.43	8.29	13.03	6.83	6-40
Psychosomatic stress reactions (W-PS)	16.54	4.95	13.81	4.02	8-39
Anxiety-state (SRQ-AS)	40.31	9.93	35.88	8.76	20-80
Use of sleeping pills and sedatives (MC-S)	.14	.34	.06	.25	0-1
Frequency of visits to the doctor (MC-D)	.88	1.36	.37	.63	( )
Pessimism about course of illness (PI)	1.31	.98	1.36	1.19	0-4
Projective measures:					
Loneliness and isolation (IBP-LI)	18.31	4.63	17.40	5.21	10-40
Anxiety and insecurity (IBP-AI)	20.35	3.58	19.73	4.42	7-28
Positive feelings (IBP-P)	17.80	2.71	17.04	3.51	6-24
Helplessness (IBP-H)	15.88	2.61	15.53	2.84	5-20
Anxiety about not being able to keep it up (IBP-AK)	6.50	1.96	5.65	1.84	3-12
Feelings of guilt (IBP-G)	4.28	1.53	3.91	1.64	2-8

( ) = unlimited scale range

Appendix VI
Correlations between the behavioral assessment scales and the problem behavior assessment scales for the parents, on the one hand, and the anxiety scales and depression scales for the children, on the other hand

VI.1 Pearson correlations >.20 between the behavioral assessment scales (BAP) for the mothers (M) and the fathers (F), on the one hand, and the anxiety and depression scales for the child, on the other hand

Anxiety and depression scales for the child	Behavioral assessment scales							
	BAP-CR		BAP-ChD		BAP-OI		BAP-NA	
	M	F	M	F	M	F	M	F
Anxiety scales:								
ST-AT	.48**	.40**	.27*					
ST-AS	.21	.26	.31*				.29*	
LAT-HP								
LAT-ITW			.22					
BLOCK-HP					.25			
BLOCK-ITW								
HP-FP			-.33*					
HP-DA	.24		.27*					
IBC-AF			.27					
Depression scales:								
DQC	.41**		.31*	.27*			.27*	
NE-se	.39**		.29*	.28*			.22	
NE-ese								
NE-f	.22			.22			.21	
HP-LI								
HP-F					.22			
HP-G								.23
IBC-LI	.35	.33	.32					
IBC-P		.29	.23	-.29			.42*	
HP-P								

* = p<.05
** = p<.01
For the abbreviatons used, see Outline of instruments, section 5.3.

VI.2 Pearson correlations >.20 between the problem behavior assessment scales (PBAP) for the mothers (M) and the fathers (F), on the one hand, and the anxiety and depression scales for the child, on the other hand

Anxiety and depression scales for the child	PBAP-SL M	PBAP-SL F	PBAP-B M	PBAP-B F	PBAP-E M	PBAP-E F	PBAP-SC M	PBAP-SC F
Anxiety scales								
ST-AT								
ST-AS								
LAT-HP								.23
LAT-ITW								.25
BLOCK-HP			.43**			.27		
BLOCK-ITW								
HP-FP								
HP-DA			.29*	.43**				
IBC-AF					.39			
Depression scales								
DQC			.32*	.25				
NE-se			.42**	.32*				
NE-ese			.21					
NE-f							.21	.22
HP-LI								
HP-F					.23			
HP-G			.22	.30*			.22	
IBC-LI						-.21		
IBC-P	.24						-.40	.56*
HP-P	-.27	-.22						

* = p<.05
** = p<.01
For the abbreviatons used, see Outline of instruments, section 5.3.

Appendix VII
Correlations between disease characteristics and emotion variables of the children and the parents

VII.1 Pearson correlations >.20 between the disease characteristics and the anxiety variables of the children

Disease variables	Anxiety variables				
	ST-AT	HP-FP	IBC-AF	LAT-ITW	BLOCK-HP
Time since diagnosis	.22				-.28*
Prognosis		.22		.21	
Diagnosis		-.27*			
Relapse/Recurrence		.35**			
1st Remission		-.34*			
In (subsequent) remission				-.23	
Treatment duration					-.23
Undergoing treatment		.31*	.26		
Frequ. visits to clinic	-.29*	.29*	.32	.28*	
Number of hospital admissions				.29*	
Number of days in hospital					
Physical-visible impairments					.32*

* = p<.05
** = p<.01

For the abbreviatons used, see Outline of instruments, section 5.3.

VII.2 *Pearson correlations >.20 between the disease characteristics and the depression variables and positive feelings of the children*

Disease variables	Depression variables and positive feelings								
	DQC	NE-se	BAP-ChD	IBC-P	IBC-LI	HP-LI	HP-F	HP-G	HP-P
Time since diagnosis	.22	.31*	.24*						.44**
Prognosis				.29	.21	.25			
Diagnosis						-.31*			
Relapse/Recurrence				.36		.47**			
1st Remission					-.26	-.31*			
In (subsequent) remission					-.21			.26	
Treatment duration	.25	.40**	.31*			.28*			.31*
Undergoing treatment						.28*			-.23
Frequ. visits to clinic						.32*		.27*	
Number of hospital admissions		.25		.27					.27*
Number of days in hospital							.27*	.22	
Physical-visible impairments	.22								.35**

* = p<.05
** = p<.01
For the abbreviatons used, see Outline of instruments, section 5.3.

VII.3 Pearson correlations >.20 between the disease characteristics and the children's negative experience of family relations (FRT)

| | Negative feelings | | | | | |
| | of the 4 to 7 year olds (n=26) | | | of the 8 to 16 year olds (n=56) | | |
Disease variables	towards mother	towards father	towards siblings	towards mother	towards father	towards siblings
Time since diagnosis			.63**	.23		
Prognosis			-.43*	.27*		-.26
Diagnosis	-.21		-.34			
Relapse/Recurrence						
1st Remission						
In (subsequent) remission	-.29		.21			.25
Treatment duration			.64**	.35**		
Undergoing treatment	.25		-.39			
Frequ. visits to clinic			-.46*		-.34*	-.21
Number of hospital admissions				.40**		-.24
Number of days in hospital				.45**		-.21
Physical-visible impairments			-.44*		-.23	

* = $p<.05$
** = $p<.01$

VII.4 Pearson correlations >.20 between the disease characteristics and the children's positive experience of family relations (FRT)

Disease variables	Positive feelings of the 4 to 7 year olds (n=26)			of the 8 to 16 year olds (n=56)		
	towards mother	towards father	towards siblings	towards mother	towards father	towards siblings
Time since diagnosis						
Prognosis			.48*			
Diagnosis						
Relapse/Recurrence						
1st Remission						
In (subsequent) remission						
Treatment duration						
Undergoing treatment						.24
Frequ. visits to clinic	.21		.42*			-.23
Number of hospital admissions			.25		.29*	
Number of days in hospital						
Physical-visible impairments			.27			

* = p<.05

VII.5 Pearson correlations >.20 between the disease characteristics and the assessment of the child's behavioral problems by the mother (n=81)

Disease variables	Behavioral problems				
	BAP-CR	BAP-OI	PBAP-B	PBAP-E	PBAP-SC
Time since diagnosis	.21				
Prognosis		-.21			
Diagnosis					-.22
Relapse/Recurrence					.30*
1st Remission					-.33**
In (subsequent) remission		-.27*			-.43**
Treatment duration	.21				.26*
Undergoing treatment				.21	.25*
Frequ. visits to clinic					.24*
Number of hospital admissions			.26*		
Number of days in hospital					
Physical-visible impairments			.33**		.26*

* = p<.05
** = p<.01
For the abbreviatons used, see Outline of instruments, section 5.3.

VII.6 Pearson correlations >.20 between the disease characteristics and the assessment of the child's behavioral problems by the father (n=78)

Disease variables	Behavioral problems					
	BAP-CR	BAP-OI	PBAP-SL	PBAP-B	PBAP-E	PBAP-SC
Time since diagnosis						
Prognosis						
Diagnosis			-.25*			-.23
Relapse/Recurrence						.21
1st Remission						
In (subsequent) remission		-.22				-.21
Treatment duration			.24*			.31*
Undergoing treatment					.24*	
Frequ. visits to clinic	-.21					
Number of hospital admissions						
Number of days in hospital			.22	.31**		.22
Physical-visible impairments				.21	.22	

* = p<.05
** = p<.01
For the abbreviatons used, see Outline of instruments, section 5.3

VII.7 Pearson correlations >.20 between the disease characteristics of the child and the emotion variables of the mothers (n=81)

Disease variables	Emotion variables				
	W-P	W-PS	SRQ-AS	PI	IBP-LI
Time since diagnosis					.32**
Prognosis				.21	
Diagnosis				-.29**	
Relapse/Recurrence		.22		.27*	
1st Remission				-.21	
In (subsequent) remission					
Treatment duration	.24*	.34**		.34**	.22
Undergoing treatment					-.24*
Frequ. visits to clinic			.21		
Number of hospital admissions		.26*			
Number of days in hospital	.22*	.28*			
Physical-visible impairments					-.24*

* = p<.05
** = p<.01
For the abbreviatons used, see Outline of instruments, section 5.3

VII.8 *Pearson correlations >.20 between the disease characteristics of the child and the emotion variables of the fathers (n=78)*

Disease variables	Emotion variables						
	W-PS	SRQ-AS	MC-S	PI	IBP-P	IBP-AK	IBP-G
Time since diagnosis	.26*						
Prognosis							
Diagnosis							
Relapse/Recurrence		.22	.33**		-.35**		
1st Remission			-.30**			.25*	.21
In (subsequent) remission		-.21	-.30**	.26*			
Treatment duration		.34**	.22				
Undergoing treatment	-.22				-.23*		
Frequ. visits to clinic				.23*			
Number of hospital admissions			.21				
Number of days in hospital							
Physical-visible impairments			.25*				

* = p<.05
** = p<.01
For the abbreviatons used, see Outline of instruments, section 5.3.